spa magic

spa magic

CREATE A SPA AT HOME—WITH HEALING,
REJUVENATING, AND BEAUTIFYING RECIPES
FROM SPAS AROUND THE WORLD

mary muryn

A Perigee Book

Reflexology charts are from the bestselling book
Feet First: A Guide to Foot Reflexology written by Laura Norman.

A Perigee Book
Published by The Berkley Publishing Group
A division of Penguin Putnam Inc.
375 Hudson Street
New York, New York 10014

First edition: December 2002

Visit our website at www.penguinputnam.com

Library of Congress Cataloging-in-Publication Data

Muryn, Mary.
    Spa magic / by Mary Muryn.
        p. cm.
    Includes index.
    ISBN 0-399-52823-7
    1. Baths, Warm—Therapeutic use.   2. Beauty, Personal.   3. Healing.
    4. Aromatherapy.   I. Title.

RM822.W2 M867   2002
613'.4—dc21

                                                2002025127

Printed in the United States of America

10 9 8 7 6 5 4 3 2

To my mother, Anna Muryn,
who knew that beauty is a gift
a woman gives to herself.

CONTENTS

ACKNOWLEDGMENTS

I would like to thank those who were part of the journey and vision of *Spa Magic*:

Sari Botton, whose talents as a writer and editor brought this book to life

Linda Cahan, for her many years of friendship and support in all my projects

Jill Grinberg, my agent, for believing in *Spa Magic*

Cathy Cash, who started me on my journey as a writer

Van and Dianne Berhard, on whose private island in the Bahamas the vision of this book first manifested

Gerie Bauer of Great Spas of the World, International Health Spa Specialists, for making arrangements with the spas and steering me in the right direction

Julia Gajcak, for her friendship and support

Joan Ruggiero, who did the hard part—keeping things organized and on track

Charlie Karp, who was a great sport experimenting with the unknown when it came to our spa adventures in remote places

Maya Meguro, for initiating me into the art of the Japanese bath

Sheila Curry Oakes, my editor at Perigee, for giving this book a home.

INTRODUCTION

*I*magine going to an exotic spa every day, rejuvenating your body, mind, and spirit with aromatherapy, scrubs, facials, reflexology massages, and other luxurious treatments while unwinding to meditative music in beautiful, soothing surroundings. While it sounds wonderful, it probably also sounds incredibly decadent—not to mention expensive and impossible. But that's not the case at all.

In fact, it is possible to have world-class spa experiences daily, right in your own home, without spending a lot of money. What's more, those treatments, once thought to be mere indulgences, are actually important to maintaining optimal health and emotional well-being. They restore harmony and balance to the body by stimulating the body's circulatory, lymphatic, and elimination systems, ultimately helping to release the toxins and stress that build up in our bodies and minds. Physical balance and emotional harmony are the foundations of good health—which in turn is the foundation of beauty.

Take care of yourself this way, and feel your heart lighten, watch the stress lines in your face begin to fade, and see your complexion begin to glow.

You *need* to take time out each day to escape and reconnect peacefully to your inner self—to take care of your being at every level—in order to be at your best and to do your best in all the areas of your life, and to fulfill your dreams. It is vital to release all that stands in the way of your well-being: pain, frustration, and negativity. A few minutes even on hectic days can make a difference. Your morning shower can easily incorporate an aromatic, homemade body scrub. There are quick, simple treatments you can administer in your office, designed to revive you while at work.

What I want to give you in this book—beyond recipes and instructions for treatments from the world's best spas—is permission to take time to nurture and pamper yourself, as well as a new perspective on your health. I want to show you that you needn't feel guilty for taking care of yourself with spa treatments. When you nurture yourself, you will be better equipped to nurture those around you. I also want to help you get more comfortable with the concept of self-love, a key component to wellness. Creating the space in your life to give yourself rejuvenating, healing treatments requires an attitude of self-love, which in itself is healing. The practices you adopt—from the simplest to the most elaborate—will support and enhance your well-being even more, helping you to feel *and look* your best.

Our state of mind, our health, and our physical appearance are all connected. Our emotions can often be read not only in our facial expressions but also in our physical condition. Emotional stress, which can contribute to and exacerbate all illness, is reflected in any medical conditions we might have. There are very specific correlations between certain stored emotions and particular manifestations in sickness.

So many of us get accustomed to storing and swallowing stress and negativity without even realizing their toll on us. This way of living comes to feel normal. The treatments in this book will help you to remove those harsh feelings and their attendant ailments. Cleanse your pores, and open the gateway to cleansing your soul. Relax your mind, and watch your skin clear up. Once you begin to adopt some of the practices I offer, it won't be long before you notice that you feel better, inside and out.

I've had so many positive experiences with spa treatments, which is why they are part of my daily routine. But one experience in particular made the importance of those treatments eminently clear to me. Prior to a trip to Bali, to write an article about the spas there, I started to experience premenopausal symptoms—hot flashes, vaginal dryness, bloating, mood swings, and a lack of energy. After two weeks of massages, reflexology, aromatherapy, body scrubs, wraps, and facials, all of my symptoms were gone.

I know—as the people of much older cultures have known for centuries—that facials, body scrubs, aromatic baths, massages, and the like aren't just so much pampering. Spas are now transcending their Me Generation image as indulgence emporiums, to once again being considered healing centers, as they were in ancient times. In fact, the word *spa* is a Latin acronym for *solus per acqua,* which translates to "healing by water." Our culture is coming around to the age-old wisdom that in order to look good, you need to feel good—and vice versa: looking good can actually help to make you feel good, too. In order to be healthy and radiant through and through, it is important that we incorporate restorative, cleansing, and healing practices into our everyday lives.

Now you can create a healing center in your own home, with the recipes I provide from world-class spas around the globe, along with tips on creating the right environment and learning to embrace self-love. Most of what I share with you I have discovered in my work as a healer and writer, which has taken me around the world and allowed me to immerse myself in the ancient healing traditions of many cultures. I have researched and compiled the recipes for many wonderful treatments and rituals that have survived from the Japanese, Roman, and Greek bathhouses of antiquity, and from the apothecaries of the Chinese, Indian, Balinese, Javanese, and Native American traditions.

Many of the ancient recipes you'll find here come from some of the most famous spas in the world—like the Four Seasons, Bali and the Ojai Spa in California—which pay homage to local indigenous healing traditions in the treatments that they offer. Others come from smaller boutique spas that also draw on ancient traditions.

All are designed to help you to cleanse, heal, and nurture every aspect of your being. I have written this book to show you a path of love and healing, which should be the basis for any truly spiritual spa journey.

I invite you to discover the magical, alchemical healing properties of the recipes in this book. Don't be surprised if your life is transformed in many subtle yet profound ways, giving you a greater sense of beauty, health, and harmony.

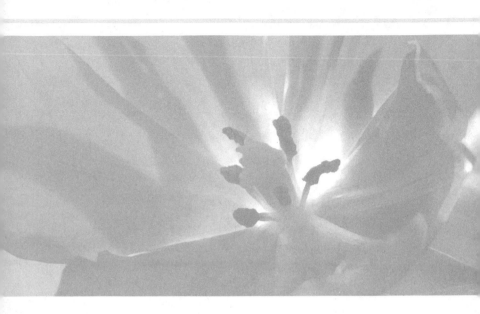

CHAPTER ONE

A Spa Primer

*R*e-creating luxurious and restorative spa experiences in your own environment can be easy to do. But it helps to have some background information so that you understand all the concepts I discuss, and so that you are able to perform the treatments in the most effective ways.

Before you begin, you'll need a basic understanding of how spa treatments work and how to make the most of them for yourself. I will explain the healing properties of water and salt water, the science of essential oils and aromatherapy, the mind/body/spirit connection, the flow of positive and negative energy throughout the body, and the body's energy centers. These are the major elements in the healing science used in spas throughout the ages. They're behind most treatments, whether they are drawn from age-old traditions or newly formulated based on ancient wisdom.

THE MIRACLE OF WATER

Water is the number-one key component to the spa experience—not to mention life on this planet. There is a great deal to be said about the magical healing, cleansing, and nourishing properties of water. In ancient Rome, France, Japan, and many other parts of the world, bathing was one of the most significant healing practices for a wide array of ailments, major and minor. There were baths for everyday health maintenance, and curative ones for times of sickness. Doctors prescribed a trip to the sea for patients, and they would go to seaside spas to "take the waters." Different herbs and oils were used to treat different maladies, often successfully. When you combine water with elements from the plant and mineral kingdoms, there is a certain mysterious, miraculous synergy that creates forces for healing.

Water is not only crucial to the spa experience—it's crucial to life. Without water, there would be no life—no humans, no animals, no plants, no food—on Earth. The Earth's surface is three-quarters water. Our bodies are 70 percent water, which is why water plays such an integral role in our health. We cleanse ourselves, inside and out, with water. When we drink water, we encourage the movement of toxins outward through our pores and our elimination system. By bathing, we cleanse ourselves from the outside in, as our bathwater penetrates our skin.

Water also facilitates the flow of energy. For this reason, one of the best places to meditate and do creative visualization is the bathtub. The water encourages the outward flow of negative energy from the body, and it also magnetizes your thoughts and intentions. Focus on positive thoughts and desires, and they will be easily manifested. Be careful not to focus on negative ones!

Drinking water also helps our brains to function more effectively. It's vital to drink a full, eight-ounce glass before a test, a meeting, or anytime you need to make a decision.

Water is truly a magical, mystical thing. It has played a role not only in physical healing, but also in spiritual cleansing for ages—two concepts that ancient cultures recognized, and we are now recognizing, to be closely linked. Water is significant in Christian Baptism. In Orthodox Judaism, there is the ritual bath, the Mikvah, used by women monthly, and by men before certain religious occasions. The Muslims have footbaths outside many of their mosques to be used before entering for prayer. In fact, the Dead Sea in Israel is a spiritual center for all three of these major religions.

SALT THAT'S GOOD FOR YOU

The Dead Sea has the highest concentration of salt of any body of water in the world. It is possible to feel weightless while floating in the Dead Sea and at the same time reap the benefits of the extreme salinity.

Saltwater is especially cleansing and healing to the body because it helps draw toxins out. Saline solution (saltwater) is very similar to our bodily fluids and our blood plasma; in a saltwater bath, the water permeates our skin, and both cleans out and replaces the toxin-filled fluids.

Thelassotherapy, one of the greatest water treatments I've experienced, is based on the therapeutic properties of sea water. Thelassotherapy was developed in the ancient spas of France, and it is still widely used throughout Europe.

I had one morning of thelassotherapy treatments at Le Meridien Hotel and Spa in Bali that had a profound—and slimming—

effect on me. There were three treatments: a walking course through a saltwater pool that had jets aimed at my joints to increase circulation and lymphatic drainage; a massage with saltwater jets aimed at the energy centers, or chakras, along my spine; and a hosing down with highly pressurized saltwater as I stood against a wall. Before the treatment, my shorts were too tight; afterward, they were too loose! And I felt wonderful and energized throughout—body, mind, and spirit. Simply soaking in a saltwater bath of sea salt or sea salt and essential oils can cleanse you, heal you, and trim you.

SPA TALK: A LEXICON OF HEALING

If you've never had a spa treatment, well, you're in for some big treats. But you also might not be familiar with some of the terminology that refers to the treatments themselves.

Scrub, or exfoliating scrub: In order for the skin to efficiently breathe, release toxins, and take in nutrients, we need to clear away a layer of dead skin—a process called exfoliation. There are acidic ingredients, like alpha-hydroxies, which help to soften the dead skin. But it is scrubs that are used to lift that layer and pull it away. Ingredients will vary in courseness—from softer carrot and coconut shreds to rougher coffee grinds and sea salts—depending upon how much scrubbing needs to be done.

Cleanser: A cleanser can be many different things. It can be a bar soap, a cream soap, or an alcohol-based astringent. When cleansing the face, many women find that detergent-based soap can be too harsh for the skin. If you prefer to use soap, try to find one that has vegetable oil or glycerine as its base, and that is nondrying and nonabrasive. As for astringent-type cleansers, there are many products available in day spas, health food stores, beauty shops, and better drugstores that will cleanse and exfoliate your skin while refreshing it. When a recipe calls for a cleanser, use what you like, but remember that pure and natural will be best.

Masque: A masque is similar to what its name implies. But it doesn't necessarily just cover your face, like a mask. It can be used to cover all your skin. A masque tends to be a pasty or creamy mixture that is left to sit on the skin, so as to nourish and soften it.

Wrap: Usually, there is an element of detoxification involved in wraps. A detoxifying mixture, made with ingredients that draw impurities from the skin, is applied to the body, which is then wrapped up in seaweed or towels and left to sweat for a while. But the body may also be wrapped when it is covered with a nourishing masque, to ensure absorption.

Bath: You think you've taken a bath—but wait until you've tried some of the recipes in here. They feel like a completely different experience, as you soak in water delightfully treated to nourish your mind, body, and spirit and encourage toxin elimination.

Facial: Facials are designed to deeply cleanse, rejuvenate, and nourish the face—and sometimes they call for several processes to achieve these things, one at a time. Cleansers, scrubs, and masques are all used.

Meditation: Some people get intimidated by the idea of meditation because they think they'll have to do something difficult or esoteric with their minds. Yes, in certain traditions, meditation can have different meanings. But for our purposes, it is simply letting your mind relax, and making space for your spirit. I like to think of it this way: Prayer is talking to God; meditation is listening to God, to the divine within you. It's being in an active state of listening—to your breath, your heartbeat, and your inner being. The inner peace you achieve while meditating promotes wellness of the mind and body, which promotes beauty.

Aromatherapy: Some people mistake aromatherapy for the enjoyment of lovely fragrances. They acknowledge the influence of pleasant scents on moods. For example, if you have fond memories of a rosebush in your backyard when you were growing up, the smell of roses today will automatically bring you back to the positive feelings of those times. But aromatherapy is much more than sweet smells. It is an intricate science: It is the extraction and distillation of essences of plants. Scientists have discovered that your nose—your olfactory system, really—has a direct passageway to your brain. When you inhale the fragrance of a plant or its essential oil, you take in the gaseous molecules of that plant, and that causes a series of reactions in the brain, which in turn stimulate a series of reactions throughout the body. When the molecules are inhaled or massaged into the body, they enter the bloodstream, therapeutically affecting the organs and glands of the body. Breathing in the essence of a flower or plant, you expose your brain to information that causes it to release endorphins and pheromones, which cause the rest of the body to be relaxed or stimulated, cooled or heated.

Because artificial scents don't have the right molecular structure, they don't have the same effect on the brain and the body. So, while a synthetic rose-scented oil might make you feel nostalgic for a minute or two, it won't give you the full effect of true aromatherapy, invigorating or calming your body, mind, and spirit. And you certainly won't have the antiseptic benefits. You might even have an allergic or asthmatic reaction to an artificial fragrance. Many people do.

Whenever possible, use real essential oils in the spa recipes you whip up. Look for the words "pure essential oil" when you are shopping for them in a health food store, a Spa gift shop, or through online and mail order companies found in the resource guide like www.frontierherb.com and Aromaland (1-800-AROMALAND). Yes, you can also use plant leaves and flower petals in your bathwater, body scrubs, masques, massage oils, and more.

The five elements: All Eastern Medicines share their roots with the basic theory that the body is governed by the 5 elements of ether, air, fire, water, and earth. Although there are some differences, there is a great deal of overlap among the traditions of Acupuncture, Reflexology, Ayurvedic, and Chinese Medicine. Many ancient healing traditions also incorporate the theory of the 7 Chakras as part of the body's energy system.

Chakras: All matter is energy—atoms and molecules in motion—our bodies included. In fact, energy governs our bodies, minds, and spirits and the way they operate together. The energy centers in our bodies have been described and understood differently by various cultures. The ancient Hindu Scholars, who founded Ayurvedic medicine, called them chakras, with the seven primary centers aligned along the spinal column. The elements have their place here; each body part is governed by an element, and each element is governed by the chakras. The Chinese called them meridians, with many different points throughout the body, but many acupuncturists today refer to the chakras as well. The meridian points are key to reflexology, a method of treating the entire body through points in the hands and feet. In both systems, points in the body are seen to affect the mind and internal organs in certain ways.

Because I will refer to both chakras and meridians in many of the chapters of this book, it will help to have a basic understanding of these systems.

A Guide to the Chakras

The ancient Hindus identified seven main energy centers in the body, located vertically along the spine and above it, called the chakras. Each chakra is associated with the functions of the internal organs as well as certain emotional and spiritual qualities. We can treat the rest of the body through our chakras. There's also a color associated with each chakra, which can be used, through visualization or other color therapy techniques, to heal the areas of the body that the chakras govern.

1. *The Root Chakra.* Located at the base of the spine, the root chakra connects you to the earth. This is where you get your strength and courage, and your fire. It is responsible for some of the reproductive organs in women and the prostate in men, as well as the colon and the backs of the legs in both sexes. The color associated with it is red.

2. *The Sacral Chakra.* The sacral chakra sits about two inches below the height of your navel. Here lies a great deal of the energy for sexuality, creativity, and creation. Because this chakra controls not only sexual appetite but thirst and hunger as well, this is also the chakra associated with addictions and attachments. It is associated with the

fronts of the legs, the reproductive organs, the intestines, and the lower back. The color associated with it is orange.

3. *The Solar Plexus Chakra.* The solar plexus, located at the navel, is like an energetic, radiant sun at the center of your being. This is where you get most of your energy for physical activity and your power for dealing with emotional matters. This chakra governs the abdomen, the pancreas, the spleen, the adrenal glands, the upper colon, the kidneys, and the liver. Its color is yellow.

4. *The Heart Chakra.* The heart chakra is located, appropriately, at the level of your heart. Most of our emotional sensitivity is centered here. The heart chakra is associated with the functions of the chest, the lungs, the heart, the lymphatic system, and the breasts. The color associated with it is green, but pink can also be used for healing this chakra.

5. *The Throat Chakra.* The throat chakra, located in the hollow of your neck, is responsible for your creativity and communicative skills. When you speak your mind, you do it from here. This chakra oversees the neck, the throat, the ears, the thymus, the salivary glands, the tongue, the teeth, and the lymph nodes in the neck. Its color is blue.

6. *The Third Eye Chakra.* Between and slightly above your eyebrows, you'll find your third eye chakra. This is the seat of intuition, enlightenment, and wisdom. Through this chakra you can view your past, present, and future. The third eye chakra is responsible for the head, the brain, the hypothalamus, the limbic system, the eyes, and the pituitary gland. The color associated with it is a violet-purple.

7. *The Crown Chakra.* At the top of your head, the crown chakra acts as a link between your human and spiritual

identities, your core self and your higher self. Your spirituality is based here, along with your consciousness of the universe beyond you. This chakra governs the top of the head. The color associated with it is white.

Energy Meridians

Albert Einstein's famous formula $E = mc^2$ proved that matter could be converted into energy. It also proved the existence of an inexhaustible form of energy called the life force. This life force runs through the body through channels called the five elements of ether, air, fire, water, and earth.

Ether corresponds to the head and neck and the three higher chakras. It also runs down the center of the body.

Air rules the heart and lungs and the heart chakra.

Fire governs the liver, gallbladder, stomach, and pancreas and corresponds to the solar plexus chakra.

Water is associated with the reproductive system, kidneys, and bladder and relates to the second chakra.

Earth corresponds to the first chakra, the root chakra. This gives new meaning to the expression "grounding yourself."

LOVE THE ONE YOU'RE WITH

Whether you're looking to tone your complexion with a facial, ease your mind in an aromatic bath, or detoxify and polish your skin with a body scrub, you need to begin with an attitude of gentleness toward yourself and self-love. This positive disposition can make all the difference in the world in terms of the effectiveness of the spa treatments you give yourself. It will also help you to live a happier life—and to look better! There is a certain positive glow that comes from liking yourself and treating yourself accordingly.

Self-love is something many of us lose sight of along the way. We learn to take care of others but not ourselves, and get rewarded in insignificant ways for our selflessness. Often we get tricked into thinking it's too selfish to take loving care of ourselves when we could be taking care of our children, our spouses or partners, our parents, our bosses. The truth is, we can't really be there for the other people in our lives until we're first there for ourselves.

How often do you feel burned out from tending to everyone else's needs and resentful toward those people in your life? This resentment creeps into everything you do, and into your relationships. Ultimately, no one is happy, and no one feels well. If you would just give to yourself generously, you will have plenty to give to everyone else.

Some may find the concept of self-love to be elusive. They may have a negative body image or think they're not pretty enough, which poisons their attitude toward themselves. A big part of self-love is accepting how you look, and realizing that when you love yourself, you are naturally beautiful. Beauty is not defined by society's model standards, which change all the time. Everyone is beautiful in their own, unique ways, and we radiate our beauty when we love and accept ourselves.

Finding and adopting self-love is easier than you think. It begins with telling yourself that you deserve to treat yourself well, and to create time for luxurious and healing spa treatments. The next step is to connect with your inner core, through breathing and visualization. The guided meditation below will help you to do that. Even if you have doubt, simply following this simple meditation will help you find the self-love you deserve and need.

Guided Meditation: Self-Love

To receive the full benefits from this meditation, if possible, read it softly and slowly into a tape recorder. Rewind, relax, and play the guided meditation back as you sink into a comfortable position. Turn off the phones, radio, television, and that little voice inside your head that never stops telling you what needs to be done.

Close your eyes and relax. Begin taking deep breaths. When you inhale, feel the breath filling up your nostrils, and then let it fill your entire body. Be conscious of your body from head to toe. With each inhalation, breathe deeper. Let the breath travel all the way through you, as if it could go way down to the soles of your feet, and then slowly exhale. Inhale again, let the breath travel all the way down to the soles of your feet, and exhale. Establish a gentle rhythm, inhaling deeply and then exhaling fully.

Once you've got a steady rhythm, begin to imagine that when you're inhaling, you're drawing your breath from a giant ball of white light. This ball of light is powerful and its energy transforms every cell in your body. Breathe in that pure white light.

Now, I want you to become aware of any constriction around your heart and lungs when you breathe. Take a few moments to breathe in and out of your chest. Let your chest expand with each inhalation, and then empty it all the way out. Inhale, expand the chest, exhale, contract the chest. As you repeat this, begin looking inside yourself. Can you see what it is that is tightening your heart and lungs? Is it fear? Anxiety? Is it physical or emotional pain? Or is it something that you can't put your finger on?

You'll be tempted to run away from yourself here. Don't. Stay with your heart, and look at what's there. Come as close to those uncomfortable feelings as you possibly can, and just let them be. Don't chase them away.

Now, visualize the most loving part of you—the part of you who takes care of family and friends, and who can embody a joy for life. Let that part of you embrace these uncomfortable feelings without judgment, and give you comfort enough to release the tension around your chest and heart.

Keep focusing on the image of this loving being inside yourself. In your mind, give her life, give her form, give her a voice. Take her hand, and walk side by side with her. Imagine you're strolling beside the seashore while the warm sun is beaming. You have a long stretch of beach to share only with the birds and marine life, so take as long as you want. The two of you are looking forward to a glorious new day that you'll spend together, talking and getting to know one another. This loving self inside of you, what are her passions? What are her dreams? Remember them so that you can write them down later, or paint or draw them as pictures. Get to know this part of you, intimately, and let her come into your waking life to take care of you, not just the people around you.

After you've gotten to know each other and you've walked for a while, stand face-to-face with this woman who is your most loving, inner self, and look at her eyes. Feel the connection and imagine there's a force coming from her eyes, a force of love, and it's drawing you inside of her. Allow yourself to merge with your innermost loving self, and create a place inside yourself where you feel comforted, peaceful, and joyous.

Now, as one fully integrated being, walk back along the beach, and visualize venturing into your heart chakra. See it as a great room with a beautiful golden throne, where your innermost loving self sits. See that part of you sitting there, totally at peace, offering comfort and grace to you constantly. Love yourself from this place, and realize that this is where all your power comes from. Allow feelings of power and self-love to permeate your entire body, every cell. You're energized. You feel like a small child, who is free and has no cares. Allow yourself to play, allow your mind to wander in imagination. You have no barriers. This is who you really are. You are a free and loving being, totally at peace with the universe. Stay here as long as you like, and when you're ready, open your eyes.

THE NEXT STEP

In the next chapter, I provide information on all the tools and ingredients you'll need for your spa journey. You're just about ready to get started. Thumb through the book and, depending on the type of treatment you want and the time you have available to you, choose an easier or more time-consuming treatment. Better yet, *make the time*. You need it. And you're worth it.

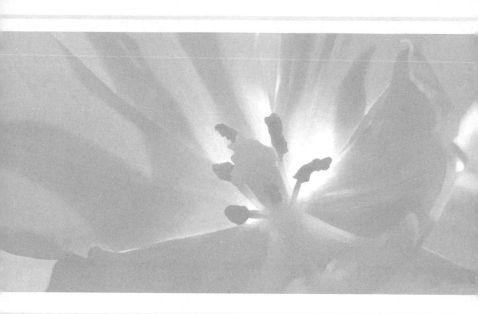

CHAPTER TWO

Getting Started

*P*erforming healing treatments from famous spas in your own home may sound a bit daunting, but it is actually quite easy and, more important, so enjoyable. Once you acquaint yourself with some of the easily found ingredients and tools of the trade, it will become second nature for you to just set aside the time you need, whip up the necessary tonics and potions, and nurture yourself from head to toe, inside and out. Here, I've put together some lists, descriptions, and explanations that will help you to get started.

EARTHLY INGREDIENTS FOR
HEAVENLY RESULTS

The big cosmetics companies may rely on chemists to create beauty formulas with highly engineered synthetic, artificial ingredients, but not you. Like the beauty specialists at the world's great spas and the ancient healers before them, you are going to use some of the most basic substances in nature to bring out your best nature.

Food items—including fruits, vegetables, herbs, spices, salts, oils, and coffee—can often feed us from the outside in, as well as the more traditional way. A good portion of the ingredients used in spa treatments can be found in the kitchen—or the supermarket or health food store.

Other basic items, like clays, muds, essential oils, and carrier oils, can be found in day spas, bath and beauty shops, and health food stores.

And don't forget to stop at the flower shop, for fresh blooms to provide aromatherapy and company while you rejuvenate yourself, and to add to some mixtures.

QUALITY CONTROL

Throughout the book, you'll find that I often recommend finding products of a certain quality or grade—using organic fruits and vegetables, flowers that haven't been sprayed with pesticides, olive oil that's been cold-pressed, candles made of beeswax or other natural ingredients, pure essential oils, etc.

While it is certainly best to use ingredients that are the most natural, and therefore best for your whole being, I don't want to stop you from diving in and trying recipes if you can only get your hands on more mainstream ingredients. If your olive oil isn't cold-pressed, and your salt isn't from the sea, but you're dying to do a salt scrub—go ahead! It will still be good for you. It is just that there are added benefits when you incorporate all-natural ingredients.

I do recommend that any heating of ingredients be done in a saucepan on the stove, rather than in a microwave. Microwave ovens change the molecular structures of ingredients, mutating their cells and depleting them of nutrients.

TOOLS OF THE TRADE

Not sure what the difference is between a loofah and a natural sponge? Don't know what kinds of bowls to use to mix ingredients? Does it make a difference? Read on.

Loofah: A dried natural vegetable that has the absorbency of a sponge but a strawlike abrasive surface that is useful for exfoliation.

Natural sea sponge: Sponges are naturally occurring in our oceans. These are the best sponges to use. They're soft and absorbent.

Mixing bowls: I like to avoid using metal mixing bowls, because the metal from the bowls can interact with certain ingredients, especially muds and clays. It's much better to use ceramic, glass, or wooden bowls, although plastic will be fine as well.

Bath pillow: Your bathtub may not be the most comfortable place to lie down for a while, but if you invest just a few dollars in an inflatable bath pillow, you may never want to get out of the tub. These are usually available at day spas, bath and body shops, and some home furnishings stores. Some are covered with terry cloth to make them even softer to the touch.

Candles: Candles may seem like frivolous accoutrements, but they're not. Some can really have a very powerful impact on the whole spa-at-home experience. But not all candles are created equal. It is best to find candles made with beeswax, vegetable wax, or another natural base, and which are scented naturally with essential oils, for the greatest aromatherapy benefit. Some people who use artificially scented paraffin candles may have allergic reactions.

An important note: Please be careful when using candles. There are certain pillar-shaped styles that can collapse and start a fire. This happened to me! And the potpourri, flower petals, or leaves that are in some candles can ignite and burn out of control. Always make sure you have your candles on a nonflammable surface, don't leave them burning unattended, and make sure you have a working smoke alarm.

Dry skin brush: At any day spa, health food store, or bath shop you can pick up one of these brushes, which you use on your skin when it is dry. Dry skin brushing exfoliates dry skin, improves blood circulation, and helps the body to move and release toxins. In fact, it's a good habit to adopt, every morning. At first, it might feel a little bit prickly, but as you get more used to it, it becomes refreshing. Brush everywhere, but always stroking toward the direction of your heart.

Spray bottle: Your local drugstore or garden shop will have simple, inexpensive spray bottles (often used to mist plants).

You'll spritz homemade skin toners and other refreshing tonics onto your skin with them.

Music: There's no rule saying you have to listen to New Age music while you beautify. You decide what kind of sounds you want to bring into your spa experience. If you want to be relaxed, try classical or soft rock. If you want to be uplifted, choose the kind of music that brings you there. Just be safe and make sure you keep the portable stereo or radio away from water sources.

Bach Flower Remedies: The homeopathic tinctures contain tiny amounts of flowers that have huge effects. They are used to heal the body from an emotional level.

FOODS FOR THE SKIN

Following are some of the food items you might find on some of the ingredient lists throughout the book, and what they're used for.

Avocado: A rich emollient with moisturizing, nourishing, and cooling properties.

Carrots: Shredded, they can be used in gentler exfoliating scrubs.

Citrus fruits: Lemons, limes, oranges, and grapefruits make refreshing astringents and cleansers.

Coconut: With its rich oil, coconut can be both exfoliating and nourishing to the skin when shredded and added to a mixture.

Coffee: Grounds are used in scrubs, to exfoliate and soften the skin, and to draw out toxins.

Cucumbers: Famous for their cooling properties, cucumbers also provide a gentle astringent.

Ginger: A stimulating, energizing root that creates heat and awakens the senses.

Honey: Honey is soothing and healing to the skin, and it gives stickiness and pliability to mixtures for masques and scrubs. Read the label—a lot of commercial honey products are filled with sugar and chemicals.

Oatmeal: Oats can be used as the basis for a gentle and soothing scrub.

Organic: When I talk about organic fruits and vegetables, I am referring to those which have been grown without pesticides, on soil which has been maintained in a healthy way, and which has not been genetically modified. Often pesticides or bad soil can undo all the benefits of otherwise healthy foods. Whenever possible, I recommend using organic produce—in your "home spa" and in your kitchen.

Salt: Salt has wonderful drawing properties, promoting the removal of toxins from the skin. It is also abrasive, which makes it a good ingredient for scrubs. But the right kind of salt, with a high mineral content, can also nourish the body. Sea salt, and salts from certain mineral-rich mines, have the highest mineral content, and so are the most nourishing. For convenience, I often recommend picking up a big box of kosher salt, which is very inexpensive. But it is best to use natural, noniodized sea salt, especially if you are treating a skin ailment.

Spices: Some of the recipes in this book call for exotic spices, like turmeric, cinnamon, cardamom, and nutmeg. You can pick these up in your local health food store, your supermarket, or order them online from resources like www.frontierherb.com.

Sugar: You won't get fat by feeding your body sugar from the outside. Sugar adds an abrasive element to scrubs, and also has healing properties on the skin.

Vinegar: The acidity of vinegar helps to break down dead skin cells so they can be easily swept away.

Yogurt: Often used as a base for masques, to cool and nourish the skin.

PLAYING IN THE MUD

Muds and clays are an essential component in many spa treatments. The two are essentially the same thing, although clay tends to have more of an elasticity to it. But both have tremendous therapeutic effects, as many cultures have known since ancient times, and can be used interchangeably.

Mud and clay have drawing properties, which assist the body in removing toxins. But they also feed the skin nutrients. Depending upon where they come from, they will have different combinations and levels of minerals.

Dead Sea mud is among the most popular types. Because of its high salt content, it is especially good at withdrawing toxins from the skin. Volcanic clay is very rich in minerals. You can get these and other muds and clays at day spas and bath and beauty shops, as well as some online and mail-order resources, like www.beautymud.com and www.deadseacosmetics4u.com.

ALL-IMPORTANT OILS

There are two basic categories of oils used in spas—carrier oils and essential oils. Both are key ingredients, used in many mixtures and formulas for all sorts of treatments.

Carrier oils: These are the oils to which essential oils are added. Carrier oils moisturize and nourish the skin while they distribute the nutrients and aromas of the plant and flower essences that have been mixed into them. Some popular carrier oils are jojoba, sesame, almond, grape seed, and olive oil.

Essential oils: Essential oils literally contain the fragrant essences of plants, flowers, roots, fruits, seeds, woods, barks, and resins. They are used in spa treatments for the amazing health benefits they offer.

The oils are derived from processes called distillation and extraction, in which the life energy and all the healing and nurturing properties of those plants and flowers used are condensed and reduced to liquid form. The oils are captured when the original plants, flowers, or fruits are heated in water, and the steam is collected and then condensed. In just a few tiny drops, you get the effects of many plants. Oils are very active, and need to be measured out carefully; in some cases, too much of a good thing can be dangerous, causing burning or itching.

Essential oils are quite powerful, and have a wide range of

healing properties. Some are calming and others are energizing; some are warming and others are cooling; some may help your mind to focus, and others may help it to empty. They can be antiviral, antibacterial, antifungal, or antiyeast—or all of the above. They can be incorporated into just about any spa treatment recipe. Some recipes call for particular oils, but you can alter them according to the effects you desire.

Essential oils in your bathtub or your body scrub, or masque, or shampoo will help to heal your body through direct contact with your skin—and through your nose. Just ahead you'll find a chart of some popular essential oils and their benefits, which will guide you in choosing which ones you might want to use in your treatments, for certain effects.

Essential Tips

Essential oils can be used in so many different ways. Add just eight to twelve drops into your bath, shampoo, scrub, liquid soap, or face and body cream, and your cleansing and moisturizing products take on a whole new fragrant, healing life.

You can also make your own body spray, to refresh yourself at any time of the day. Simply add eight to twelve drops of your favorite essential oil to a 2 oz. spray bottle full of spring water, and spritz away, whenever you need it.

Another great refresher is an essential oil face splash. All it takes is two drops of oil, placed in a basin full of cold water. Splash your face, wash your hands—and any other part of you that needs refreshing.

Essential Oils As

Mind

RELAXING
neroli
jasmine
lavender

CREATIVITY
jasmine
orange blossom
ylang-ylang

MEDITATION
sandalwood
frankincense
clove

Physical Body

WEIGHT LOSS
juniper
grapefruit
sage
basil

HEADACHES
German chamomile
peppermint
clove
eucalyptus

MUSCLE ACHES
German chamomile
lavender
nutmeg

Hair

(Add oils to shampoo: 6 drops of oil per ounce of shampoo.)

DRY HAIR
cedarwood
sandalwood
rose

OILY HAIR
rosemary
basil
ylang-ylang

NORMAL HAIR
jasmine
juniper

Facial Skin

SENSITIVE
chamomile
lavender
jasmine

MATURE
rose
neroli
sandalwood
frankincense

INFLAMED
chamomile
rosemary
lemon
aloe

Emotions

RELAXING
lavender
chamomile
sandalwood
marjoram

STIMULATING
pine
ginger
clove
patchouli
nutmeg

BALANCING
rose
jasmine
geranium
neroli

Medicinal Perfumes

Mind

CLARITY/MEMORY
lemon
eucalyptus
rosemary

DEPRESSION
rose
patchouli
ginger
orange blossom

Physical Body

INSOMNIA
chamomile
sandalwood
lavender
marjoram

PLEASURE ENHANCERS
ginger
rose
jasmine
sandalwood

Hair: (Add oils to shampoo: 6 drops of oil per ounce of shampoo.)

HAIR GROWTH
lavender
cedarwood
rosemary

DANDRUFF
lavender
rosemary
cedarwood

Facial Skin

OILY
rose
lavender
rosemary

DRY
sandalwood
chamomile
neroli
rose

ACNE
camphor
tea tree
orange

Emotions

UPLIFTING
lemon
grapefruit
ginger
peppermint
eucalyptus

GRIEF & ANGER RELEASING
lavender
marjoram
sandalwood
frankincense
orange blossom

Please note: Pregnant women usually respond well to essential oils. But I've found that in this sensitive state, it is always best to consult with a physician or holistic health practitioner before using essential oils.

CRÈMES DE LA CRÈME

Hydrating the skin is essential after spa treatments and is often part of the process of many treatments, too. Hydration, or moisturization, is achieved through oils, lotions, and creams.

We've already covered the moisturizing carrier oils—jojoba, almond, sesame, olive, and other vegetable oils. And you probably already own lotions, whether you've purchased them from the drugstore, the health food store, a beauty shop, or someplace else.

Creams are the richest of the moisturizers. Their molecules are heavier than those of oils and lotions, and so they really sink into the skin. Two of the best base creams to use are shea butter and cocoa butter. Shea butter comes from an African plant, and cocoa butter comes from cocoa beans. They are equally rich and luxurious, leaving the skin quenched and supple.

READY TO GO

Now that you've been introduced to all the things you'll need, you're ready to get started. I hope you'll enjoy all the wonderful treatments you try. I know you will.

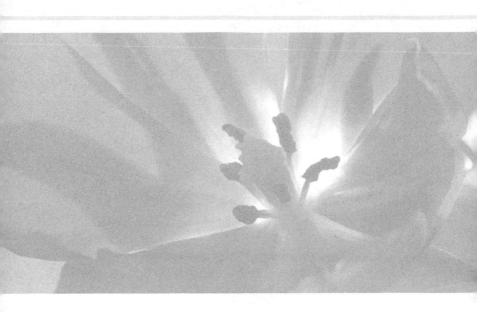

CHAPTER THREE

A Fresh Face

*I*nner peace promotes outer beauty; enhancing outer beauty fosters an internal sense of well-being, which is then radiated outward. In other words, when you feel good you look good, and when you look good, you feel good.

Treating yourself to a facial, an acupressure face massage, or a rejuvenating eye treatment can help you to achieve both. When you use time-honored ancient recipes from spas like the Four Seasons, Bali, which incorporates detoxifying natural clays, invigorating herbs, and emotionally balancing flower remedies, the toxin release, the herbal energy boost, and the homeopathic calming create a magnificent glow of inner and outer rejuvenation. I emerged from my Earth Elements Facial at the Four Seasons, Bali feeling completely relaxed and refreshed and looking years younger.

The alchemy of facials and other beauty treatments has

ancient roots. The ancient Chinese began the tradition of revitalizing the face—and the rest of the body—by massaging acupressure points on the face. Indonesian women have been giving themselves and each other facial scrubs and other treatments for ages, as a matter of daily health maintenance. It is no wonder they have some of the most beautiful complexions in the world. Centuries ago, Nostradamus discovered many of the healing properties of plants, which he used to create his own line of products for facial treatments.

READING THE FACE

The face can be very revealing. Obviously, facial expressions reveal one's mood, but it goes much deeper than that. There are some psychics who can do face fortune-telling, reading your past, present, and future through lines and creases.

Your face is truly a reflection of your physical, emotional, and spiritual state. The color of your skin signals the condition of your circulatory system. If you're pale or sallow, blood isn't moving as it should be. Bags under your eyes aren't only indicative of fatigue but also of poor circulation and lymphatic congestion— the results of stress.

Stress is the true culprit behind all our less radiant moments. Stress comes in many forms, whether it's emotional aggravation and negativity or the body trying to process and eliminate toxins, like too much sugar, alcohol, or pesticides. What you eat and how you metabolize stress will show up on your face. If you truly want to be radiant (and feel great), incorporate healthy eating and exercise and find inner peace through meditation or other spiritual endeavors—and, of course, by treating yourself to nurturing spa treatments at home.

Your face can be used as a map of the rest of your body, according to Oriental medicine. There are facial nerve endings and reflexes that are connected to internal organs, so the placement of discolorations, blemishes, or even wrinkles can indicate which systems are ailing. When you treat those areas on the face, you will also be treating those organs and systems. In fact, a facial can often be the best treatment for digestive and circulatory ailments.

By doing facial treatments, you can also access and affect the third eye chakra, located just above and between the eyebrows. This is the seat of your inner vision, and also the chakra that governs your pituitary gland and endocrine/hormonal balance.

There are many varieties of facial treatments—scrubs, cleansers, masques, face massages, acupressure, and reflexology. Different techniques and ingredients will give you different effects, from toning and cleansing to removing fine lines and lifting.

Earth Elements Facial

FROM THE FOUR SEASONS, SAYAN, BALI

Many people think of a facial as the ultimate beauty treatment. At the Four Seasons in Sayan, Bali, in the lush hillside along the Agung River, my experience with a facial transcended that of a beauty treatment.

Many of the ingredients used in this facial are gathered from the earth, such as clay and fresh herbs. As they are not processed, they maintain the powers of Mother Nature. The facialist asked me whether I wanted to relax to soothing music while she worked, but this time I chose not to, as I wanted to concentrate on the treatment itself without any outside noise.

Lying on the table, observing my body, I became aware of holding on to a conversation that I had had that morning with my assistant about various business problems that had come up. She said it was not a good week. Relaxing was a bit of a challenge. Then, suddenly, I felt gentle surges of energy flowing through the upper part of my body, down to my navel. Gently, streams of energy were shifting me into an altered state. My navel felt energized, as if that was the center of my balance of power.

Suddenly, wonderful visions began popping into my third eye, like vignettes from a movie. I experienced peace and love. This was way beyond my usual experience of relaxation, well-being, and rejuvenation! This was spiritual, a feeling of inner nourishment. A seventy-five minute facial flowed into one lasting moment in time. I definitely felt relaxed, but more, I felt in touch with my entire body. But it wasn't just my spirit that soared from this treatment. The true test of any beauty treatment is what you see when you look in the mirror.

With most facials, of course your skin feels great, but do you have to talk yourself into believing you look younger? How much younger? Well, not this time. When I looked into the mirror, I practically saw a different face staring back at me: altered, relaxed and youthful. I later learned that the Four Seasons Spa in Sayan uses Australian homeopathic flower essences in this facial, which work on balancing the chakras, as well as soothing the emotions and altering your mental state to one of total tranquility. This recipe has been adopted for home use using readily available Bach Flower Remedies. This is a holistic facial based upon the principles of balancing the "earth elements" of air, fire, water, and earth. I highly recommend it, for body and soul.

Step 1: Cleansing and Toning
Your favorite cleanser
Lavender essential oil
Mustard Bach Flower Remedy

Mix your favorite cleanser with a few drops of lavender oil and mustard Bach Flower Remedy. Cleanse and rinse your face.

Step 2: Exfoliating

½ cup aloe vera gel

Ylang-ylang essential oil

Star of Bethlehem Bach Flower Remedy

Mix ingredients and massage gently into skin. Remove with a warm, moist towel.

Step 3: Steaming the Face

Bowl of almost boiling water

Sandalwood essential oil

Centaury Bach Flower Remedy

Put the oil in the water. Drape a large towel over your head and let your face absorb the steam for five or ten minutes. Pat your face with a damp compress, which has been dipped in water to which you've added five drops Centaury Bach Flower Remedy.

Step 4: Clay Masque

¼ cup of the following:

Dead Sea mud

Clay or mud masque available in the cosmetics department of a
    pharmacy or department store

1 tablespoon aloe vera gel

Your favorite essential oil

Hornbeam Bach Flower Remedy

Mix the mud and aloe vera with the hornbeam Bach Flower Remedy. Scent the mixture with a few drops of your favorite essential oil for additional nourishment for your skin. Apply to face and leave on for about ten minutes. Remove with warm towel.

Step 5: Moisturize

Chamomile essential oil

Your favorite moisturizer

Shea butter

Essential oil of your choice

Add three drops of chamomile essential oil to your moisturizer and apply it to your face. Add two drops of your choice of essential oil to a bit of shea butter, and apply to your lips.

Note: bergamont and citrus essential oils can sometimes react with the UV rays of the sun and should not be used.

DELAYED REWARDS

As you may already know, sometimes we don't look our best right after a treatment like a facial. At some spas, they put pressure on the skin to clean the pores, which creates blemishes. You're not going to do that using the recipes in this book. But some of the scrubs can be somewhat abrasive, and can draw toxins to the surface of your skin initially. Sometimes, when you begin to detoxify, impurities have a hard time finding their way out, and may cause pimples or rashes. This is not a sign that you have failed; quite the opposite—you're on your way. In a day or two, your skin will look great. And if you keep up these practices, and live more healthily, there will be less and less toxic

Bach Flower Remedies and Australian Flower Remedies Based on the Earth Elements

	Air	Fire	Water	Earth
Bach	• star of Bethlehem	• centaury	• mustard	• hornbeam
Australian	• white eromophilia • purple eromophilia	• red beak orchid • pink trumpet	• purple nymph • the goddess grasstree	• purple ename orchid • red or green kangaroo paw
Purpose	*Overcomes mental paralysis*	*Maintains drive and dynamism*	*Overcomes vulnerability and sensitivity*	*Stimulates consistency and stability*

material to work its way out. Of course, if you have a big event or meeting that you need to look good for, you shouldn't detoxify the night before. Plan to do it at least two nights before the scheduled event or meeting, or wait until afterwards.

Avo-Beta Cream Masque

FROM THE OAKS AT OJAI, OJAI, CALIFORNIA

Ojai is a lively artistic community nestled in northern Ventura County, a ninety-minute drive from Los Angeles. The Oaks at Ojai is nestled in the heart of town and offers a serene, yet upbeat atmosphere in which to get fit or pampered. "The staff at Ojai focus on creating positive healthy habits and educat-

ing guests to implement lifestyle changes," says owner/founder Sheila Cluff. In addition to treatment from the inside out, guests are pampered with massages and cleansing facials.

The combination of carrot (high in beta-carotene and antioxidant vitamins), heavy cream (high in calcium and protein), and avocado (a rich source of vitamin E) in this facial mask will improve skin texture, diminish age spots, and rebuild skin collagen when used with regularity. Egg will tighten the pores.

¼ cup heavy cream

1 carrot, cooked and mashed

1 avocado, peeled, pitted, and mashed

3 tablespoons honey

1 egg, beaten

Combine ingredients in a bowl and spread over face and neck. Relax for fifteen minutes. Rinse with cold water.

The thicker the consistency of the masque, the more intense the action on the skin.

Refresher Facial

FROM THE MANDARA SPA AT IBALY, UBUD, BALI

The Balinese believe the gods live in the mountains, and the spa setting for treatments at the Chedi reflects a feeling of sacredness and inner nourishment.

My experience at the Chedi was transcendental. I chose the Ultimate Spa

Indulgence Package. This started with an aromatherapy footbath followed by a lavender body wash and then a soothing coconut scrub. *This session was completed by a two-person massage followed by a refresher facial and a simultaneous session of reflexology—two and one-half hours of bliss!*

Step 1: Cleansing and Toning

Your favorite cleanser

Your favorite toner

Washcloth or cotton squares

Cleanse the face with your favorite cleanser using small circular strokes. Remove with warm washcloth or dampened cotton squares. Apply gentle pressure to your face as you do so. Use toner appropriate to your skin type.

Step 2: The Masque

2 tablespoons collagen powder or
cosmetic clay (available at health
food stores and spa boutiques)

1 tablespoon cucumber juice for oily
skin or carrot juice for normal to dry
skin

2 cucumber slices for eyes

Mix collagen powder (or cosmetic clay powder) together with the cucumber or carrot juice to make a paste. Apply masque with your fingers or a brush and place the cucumber slices on your closed eyes. Leave on for fifteen minutes. Gently wipe off the masque with a natural sponge or warm washcloth.

Step 3: Acupressure Massage

The face, head, and neck contain nerve centers and reflex points corresponding to your entire body. When you give yourself or receive a facial or face massage, you will also derive many other benefits, such as:

Stress relief
Increased energy
Clearer eyesight
Improved digestion
A more relaxed and youthful face

Use the middle fingers on both sides of the face simultaneously. Do two rounds—for the first use medium pressure and hold each point for five counts; the second time use lighter pressure and hold for three counts.

POINT 1	Hairline (in line with pupils)
POINT 2	Mid forehead (in line with pupils)
POINT 3	Above the midpoint of eyebrows
POINT 4	Below the midpoint of eyebrows
POINT 5	Orbital ridge (in line with pupils)
POINT 6	Sides of nose
POINT 7	Sides of mouth
POINT 8	Above midpoint of jawbone
POINT 9	Above jawbone, one inch from #8
POINT 10	Under the chin

POINT 11/12	Top and bottom midpoint of jawbone
POINT 13	Midpoint in front of ears
POINT 14	Temples
POINT 15	Cheeks (straight line down from #14)

Step 4: Moisturizing

Finish by applying your favorite moisturizer (scented with a few drops of your favorite essential oil, if you wish).

Vital Energy Eye Treatment

FROM THE CHIVA-SOM INTERNATIONAL HEALTH RESORT, HUA HIN,
THAILAND "CHIVA-SOM" TRANSLATES TO HAVEN OF LIFE.
THIS HEALTH RESORT CONTAINS ALL THE INGREDIENTS OF A MAGICAL
ELIXIR FOR PERSONAL TRANSFORMATION.

WHAT YOU'LL NEED:

Make-up Remover

Facial Cleanser

Lightweight Eye Cream

Revitalizing Eye Mask or substitute 2 Chamomile Tea Bags or
   Cucumber Slices

Eye Lotion

Eye Pads

Stressed eyes appear puffy, irritable, and sensitive and are often aggravated by modern living. Combat these effects with this calming eye treatment to soothe, refresh, and revitalize tired eyes.

1. Begin by removing your eye make-up and lipstick with eye make-up remover and then cleanse the entire face.

2. Apply a lightweight eye cream to the entire eye area, using enough product to provide "slip" from the hairline to the cheeks.

Follow the steps for this revitalizing pressure point massage, repeating each movement three times.

3. Use a Revitalizing Eye Mask to cover your eyes and relax for a few minutes or Chamomile Tea Bags or Cucumber slices, followed by cotton pads soaked in Soothing Eye Lotion, and lie back and relax for ten to fifteen minutes.

Remove eye pads and complete the treatment by applying a moisturizing eye cream.

YOGA FOR YOUR FACE

In addition to facial treatments, there are exercises you can do to rejuvenate your complexion while also treating the organs associated with certain points on your face. They come from the ancient practice of yoga. Try some of these. It will be like having a face-lift from the inside, while also helping you relax and ease your mind. These exercises have been keeping people in India and other places in the Far East looking young for centuries.

You can do these exercises quickly, spending just a few moments or seconds on each. In less than twenty minutes, you

Eye Treatment Pressure Point Massage

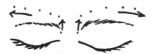

1. Using index and middle fingers, slowly press and release points from the eyebrow to the hairline. Repeat to cover the entire forehead.

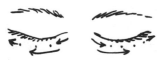

2. Apply pressure using the middle finger under the eye from the inner eye to the temple.

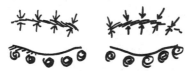

3. Pinch and press with your index finger and thumb along the eyebrow toward the temple. Next, use the middle finger and make gentle circles under the eye from the temple to the inner eye.

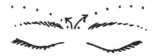

4. Apply deep pressure with your thumbs to the middle of the eyebrows. Slide your thumbs to the hairline and apply pressure along the hairline to the temples.

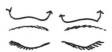

5. Using flat palms, slide up from your eyebrows to your hairline and finish with pressure at the temples.

can revitalize your face, release stress and tension from your facial muscles, and feel better for the rest of the day and night.

While it's best to do these exercises with a clean face, if you are in the office and already wearing makeup, go ahead and do the exercises anyway.

Face Calisthenics

Relax in corpse pose, flat on your back with your palms up. Try to keep your mouth closed so you breathe through your nose, and keep your tongue resting on the roof of your mouth. Relax every part of your face. Be aware of tension or stress in your face. Bring breath to any tightness in the muscles of the face, mouth, jaw, forehead, nose, head, scalp, and skin. Be aware of any holding or clenching, and release.

Imagine that you are breathing in pure, healing energy to your face and breathing out any negative energy. Let your exhaled breaths leave you completely. Relax everything.

Then, tighten isolated areas of the face, hold for a few moments, release, and relax. Next, scrunch up your whole face tightly toward your nose—forehead, mouth, eyes, cheeks. Hold for a few moments, then release and relax.

Do this for a minimum of ten minutes. Rushing through this exercise won't deliver the best results.

Lion Pose

Kneel, resting your buttocks on your heels, with your hands on your knees in front of you. Arch your back without hyperextending, keeping your head and face straight and facing forward. Widen your eyes, look up, and stick your tongue out as far as it can go.

This takes about two to three minutes.

The Rubdown

Make sure your hands are clean. Begin by rubbing the palms of your hands together vigorously. Then press your palms against your face so that you feel the warmth in your hands enter into your skin and penetrate into your facial muscles. Use your imagination and feel the energy being absorbed by the cells throughout your face. Then move your hands in an outward circular action around the face. Work the fingers and palms up through the bridge of the nose, through the third eye, and out across the forehead, proceeding down the temples and cheeks and across the chin and mouth, crossing back up along the nose. Continue to rub for as long as you feel comfortable. You may want to stop occasionally to rub your hands together, to bring more heat and energy into your face. Practice this exercise whenever your facial muscles become tired. This will help to reduce the formation of wrinkles on the skin and bring a glow to your complexion.

This exercise may be done at home or at work (if you have a private space). It will take a minimum of three minutes—but rub for as long as it feels good to do so.

Rapid Eye Movement

Sit comfortably in a cross-legged position. Relax and extend the spine upward without hyperextending. Drop your shoulders away from your ears. Bring your breath into your belly. Keeping your head straight ahead and your neck and shoulders relaxed, close your eyes and relax them. Then open your eyes and look straight up, without moving your head or scrunching your forehead, and hold. Repeat, looking down. Don't strain your eyes. Be gentle. Repeat looking up and down a few times, then rub your palms together, creating heat, and gently hold your warmed hands over your closed eyes, relaxing them and bringing healing warmth to the backs of the eyes and the eye muscles.

Repeat the same exercise, looking slowly from side to side. Then repeat the same exercise looking all around as if the eyes are the hands of a clock. Repeat in both directions slowly and gently. Rub the palms together once again and hold over the eyes, relaxing any tension and reviving tired or strained eye muscles. Uncover the eyes, and relax.

This exercise should take three to five minutes.

Fresh Fruit Facial

FROM THE NOELLE SPA FOR BEAUTY AND WELLNESS,

STAMFORD, CONNECTICUT

This premiere day spa offers water treatments, exotic facials and other European inspired treatments. "Escape to It All" has become the catchphrase for the varied internationally based spa services that can be experienced without traveling around the world. The sensitive use of feng shui principles creates an environment of energetic movement balanced with total serenity.

The Fresh Fruit Facial is designed for people who are sensitive to chemicals and preservatives in many of today's facial products. This facial is composed of only 100 percent all-natural ingredients.

FOR CLEANSING AND TONING

½ teaspoon avocado oil

3 drops lemon juice or orange juice for oily skin

Combine and rub gently into the skin with your fingertips. Remove with a warm, wet washcloth.

FOR EXFOLIATING

OATMEAL SCRUB

½ cup milk

Corn flour or oatmeal to make a paste

1 teaspoon honey

Combine ingredients, apply to face, and gently press and release. Leave on until dry. Rub off gently with a warm washcloth. This mixture allows for deep cleaning of the skin without being abrasive. The oats provide particles to remove dead skin cells, and the gentle acids found in milk and honey add additional exfoliation.

FOR OILY SKIN

½ orange (cut an orange in half crosswise)

Gently rub the cut side of the orange half onto the skin. The fruit acids will help to clean and exfoliate the skin.

FOR MASSAGE

1 teaspoon avocado oil

This is great for all skin types.

MASQUE FOR NORMAL TO DRY SKIN

1 medium banana

1 cup evaporated milk

Mash the banana and blend with the milk.

Apply the mixture to your skin with your fingers. Wrap your face with gauze.

Leave on for 15 minutes, then rinse with warm water.

Cool As a Cucumber

At the Ritz Carlton in Bali, I learned a little trick. You can treat yourself to a very quick facial rejuvenation with just a cucumber, a towel, and some lemon or lime. Slice the cucumber thinly and apply to your face while lying down. After you've relaxed with the slices on your face for about fifteen minutes, further tone your skin by squirting lemon or lime juice onto a damp towel, and then dab your face gently with it. You'll feel—and look—cool and refreshed.

MASQUE FOR NORMAL OR SENSITIVE SKIN

½ cup chamomile tea, cooled

Enough powdered milk to make a paste

Apply paste to your face with your fingers. Wrap your face with gauze. Let it dry. Remove with a warm, wet washcloth.

FOR NORMAL TO OILY SKIN

8 orange slices

Avoiding your eyes and the area surrounding them, wrap the slices of orange onto your face with gauze, and lie down for fifteen minutes. Remove gauze and oranges and rinse face with warm water.

The following chart will help you choose the right ingredients for your facial:

	Normal skin	Dry Skin	Oily Skin	Sensitive Skin
Cleanse & Tone	Avocado oil*	Avocado oil	Avocado oil mixed with a few drops of avocado and orange	Avocado oil mixed with a few drops of lemon or orange juice
Exfoliate	Instant oatmeal mixed with a touch of honey, green tea, and a splash of milk	See Oatmeal Scrub recipe.	Use Oatmeal Scrub, or for extremely oily skin, a peeled half orange gently rubbed into the skin will further deep-clean and exfoliate.	See Oatmeal Scrub recipe (page 53).
Massage	Avocado oil	Avocado oil	Avocado oil mixed with a few drops lemon or orange juice	Avocado oil with a few drops of pure rose or lavender oil
Masque**	Mix ½ banana and one strawberry with powdered milk. Add a splash of green tea. Apply to face, cover with gauze, and relax for 15 minutes.	Smash one small banana and blend with powdered milk. Apply to face and cover with gauze. Relax for 15 minutes.	Mash several fresh strawberries and mix with powdered milk and a splash of green tea. Cover with gauze and relax for 15 minutes. Or take a few slices of orange and place them on the skin. Hold them in place with gauze.	Mix powdered milk with chamomile tea. Wrap with gauze and relax with mask for 15 minutes.
Moisturize	Avocado oil	Avocado oil	Avocado oil	Avocado oil with a few drops of pure rose or lavender oil

*We recommend avocado oil because it is great for all skin, especially for anyone who has a nut allergy. If you are not allergic to nuts, you can also try almond oil. Extra-virgin olive oil is also a great oil to try.

**For a special eye treat while masquing, use the tea bags you used to make the green or chamomile tea as eye compresses. Let them cool before placing them on the eye area. Another idea is to apply slices of cucumber to the eye area.

You can make your own toner by mixing two ounces of juice from any of the following with one ounce of spring water:

Pineapple
Cucumber
Carrot
Aloe vera
Tomato

Mix thoroughly. Put in a spray bottle and use as needed.

FRESH FROM THE FRIDGE

Who needs chemical alpha-hydroxies in a bottle when you can get natural, more effective ones by just rubbing orange slices on your face? The key to a beautiful complexion could be closer than you think—right in your kitchen. You can make scrubs, cleansers, and masques for your face, and the rest of your skin, using different foods and plants.

Luciana Stanciu is an esthetician at the Noelle Spa in Connecticut. In her native Romania, she learned how to use common foods and plants to make facial scrubs, cleansers, masques, and other tonics. She offers these guidelines:

Aloe Vera (emollient, healing, soothing): Snip about an inch off of an aloe vera leaf and rub the juice into the skin.

Avocado (emollient, nourishing; especially good for mature skin): Smash up the pulp of one avocado and rub it all over the skin. Let it dry before rubbing it off and washing.

Banana (nourishing, soothing): Mash a banana and rub it onto the skin. Let it dry before rubbing off and washing.

Cantaloupe (emollient, astringent): Mash one cup of pulp and rub it into skin. Leave on for a few minutes, then wash off.

Carrot (nourishing, gently exfoliating): Mash and grate one raw carrot and rub it onto skin. Leave on for several minutes before rubbing off and then washing.

Cornmeal Flour (exfoliant and emollient): Mix one teaspoon of fine cornmeal with cooled chamomile tea to form a gentle scrub. Let dry, then gently rub off. Not for sensitive skin.

Cucumber (cooling, hydrating, whitening, astringent): Peel and mash a cucumber and use it as a masque. Leave on for several minutes, then wash off.

Egg Yolk (nourishing, lifting, tightening): Mix one egg yolk with one teaspoon of honey and rub all over the face. Let dry, then wash.

Honey (nourishing): Mix with any fruit or vegetable to make a nourishing masque.

Lemon (astringent, whitening, toning): Add a few drops of lemon juice to any masque.

Milk (emollient, exfoliant, nourishing): Make an exfoliating paste using chamomile tea and powdered milk. Rub on skin, let dry, and then rub off before washing.

Orange (astringent, exfoliant, whitening, toning): Add one teaspoon of orange juice to any masque. Or rub orange slices onto your skin as a toner.

Papaya (exfoliant, nourishing with digestive proteins): Rub slices on the skin. Not for sensitive faces.

Peach (nourishing and toning): Mash peach pulp into a masque. Rub it on, let it set for a few minutes, and rub off.

Potatoes (anti-inflammatory—great for bags under eyes!): Cover each eye with a slice of potato, and rest for fifteen minutes.

Strawberries (astringent, nourishing with vitamin C): Make a masque of mashed strawberries.

Tomatoes (astringent): Rub slices onto the skin.

Watermelon (hydrating, cooling, astringent): Rub slices onto the skin.

Yogurt (emollient, astringent, soothing): Mix two tablespoons of yogurt with one teaspoon of honey for a soothing masque.

Honey Papaya Facial

FROM KALANI SPA, PATTOA, HAWAII

This spa's unique environment includes nearby thermal springs and natural steam baths. It specializes in such natural forms of healing as Watsu, Cranio-Sacral Therapy, and Reiki.

When your skin needs a deep moisturizing treatment, this facial is great! Try it after too much sun or in the dead of winter to add a glow to your skin. Papaya is a mild exfoliant and, combined with honey, has skin-softening properties.

TONER

1 cool papaya, sliced and/or slightly mashed

Apply all over your face. Leave on for one to two minutes. Remove with a damp washcloth.

MASQUE

½ cup honey

10 drops of your favorite essential oil

Rose, lavender, jasmine, neroli, and ylang-ylang are great oils to choose for this simple masque. Mix the oil in the honey and apply to your face. Leave on for five to fifteen minutes. Wash off thoroughly with a gentle cleanser.

Special Care for Acne

FROM THE MANDARA SPA AT ROYAL GARDEN RESORT,

HUA HIN, THAILAND

A completely natural outdoor spa located on an expansive sandy beach, this is a perfect place to enjoy some of Thailand's best beauty treatments.

The Mandara Spa staff offers the following advice on the very troublesome problem of acne.

Acne is a problem that can affect anyone beyond the age of puberty. An eruption of pimples is more common in people with oily skin, especially during periods of emotional disharmony. Even the person with the finest complexion, however, is likely to experience the occasional outbreak of pimples. To avoid outbreaks, try the following:

Eat five varied portions of fruit and vegetables daily. Ideally these should be organic. Fruits and vegetables contain antioxidants, which promote clear skin and good health. If it is not possible to obtain organic, make sure to wash (and, where appropriate, peel) all fruits first.

Drink 1 cup of warm spring water

QUICKIE:
Exfoliating Skin Masque

This is an easy recipe, using foods you're likely to have around the kitchen. It's a masque that is full of the natural alpha-hydroxy acids found in commercial skin creams, which act as a gentle exfoliant to prevent the buildup of sebum. Oatmeal has a soothing effect on irritated blotchy skin.

- 1 tablespoon finely ground oatmeal
- 1 tablespoon plain live yogurt
- ¼ apple, freshly grated
- 2 tablespoons fresh lemon juice

Mix the oatmeal and the yogurt into a paste. Add the apple and lemon juice and stir well. Apply to clean dry skin and relax for fifteen to twenty minutes before rinsing off with warm water and patting the skin dry.

each morning before or after breakfast to flush out your system and help prevent constipation.

Cleanse your skin twice daily using a gentle, soap-free cleansing bar.

To dry out a troublesome isolated pimple, dab with undiluted calendula tincture or full-strength tea tree oil. Apply the tincture with a cotton bud, being careful to avoid the surrounding skin.

To subdue a cluster of pimples, try one of the following aromatic treatments:

FACIAL SAUNA FOR CONGESTED SKIN

Most skins benefit from a deep-cleansing steam treatment once or twice a week, especially congested or oily skin that is prone to pimples and blackheads.

Begin by cleansing your skin as you normally do.

Heat-proof mixing bowl filled with near-boiling water
3 drops of any of the following essential oils: either singularly or
    combined: lavender, tea tree, frankincense, juniper berry,
    lemongrass, or rosemary

Add the oil to the water. Hold your head over the steam and cover your head and the bowl with a towel to trap in the aromatic vapors. For the full benefits, stay there for about five minutes. Afterwards, splash your face with tepid water to remove wastes accumulated on the skin's surface.

For added benefit, use the following face masque after your facial sauna:

DEEP-CLEANSING CLAY MASK

This combination of green clay, yogurt, and frankincense has a deep-cleansing antiseptic and anti-inflammatory action on the skin, and is perfect for troublesome complexions. For best results, apply once or twice a week, immediately after a facial sauna, while the skin is still warm and moist and, therefore, more receptive to whatever is applied to it.

3 level teaspoons fine green clay
3 teaspoons live, organic yogurt (unflavored)
1 drop frankincense essential oil

Mix the ingredients together to form a smooth paste. Smooth over your face and throat, avoiding the delicate eye area. Leave on for ten to twenty minutes, then rinse off with tepid water. Allow the skin to settle for about one hour before applying a light moisturizer such as unscented aloe vera gel.

Special Care for Dry Skin

FROM THE IMPERIAL MANDARA SPA AT THE IMPERIAL QUEEN'S PARK,
BANGKOK, THAILAND

There is a strong philosophy at this spa that beauty is a holistic concept that embraces the inner and outer self: "Outer beauty comes from regular and ritualistic processes that use natural products for the skin."

Dry skin needs nourishment! The following recipes will enhance your skin's ability to retain moisture. In order to prevent your skin from becoming too accustomed to one product, and therefore less responsive to its therapeutic effects, it is beneficial to alternate application.

ROSE PETAL SKIN CREAM

¼ ounce beeswax granules (or grated beeswax if using a block)

1 ounce sweet almond oil

1 ounce distilled water or rosewater

3 (500mg) capsules evening primrose oil, emptied

1 ounce rosehip seed oil

5 drops rose essential oil

Put the beeswax and almond oil into the top of a double boiler.

Warm the distilled water on the stove. Remove before it boils.

Stir the beeswax and oil mixture continuously until the beeswax has dissolved. Remove from heat and transfer the mixture into a nonmetal bowl. Add the evening primrose oil (pierce the capsules with a pin and squeeze the contents into the mixture) and rosehip seed oil and stir well.

Add the distilled water to the bowl, a teaspoon at a time, while beating with a rotary whisk or electric mixer set at the lowest speed.

Continue beating until the cream begins to thicken, then stir in the rose essential oil.

Spoon the mixture into little glass pots with tight-fitting lids. This cream should be refrigerated after a few days.

ORANGE BLOSSOM SKIN CREAM

¼ ounce beeswax granules (or grated beeswax if using a block)

1 ounce cocoa butter

1½ ounces sweet almond oil

1 ounce distilled water or orange flower water

5 drops neroli essential oil

Put the beeswax, cocoa butter, and sweet almond oil into the top of a double boiler.

Warm the distilled water in another pan.

Stir the beeswax, cocoa butter, and oil mixture continuously until the beeswax has completely dissolved. Remove from the heat and slowly add the warmed distilled water, a teaspoonful at a time, while beating with a rotary whisk or electric mixer set at the lowest speed.

Continue beating until the cream begins to cool and thicken, then stir in the neroli essential oil.

This cream should be refrigerated after a few days.

Apply the Rose Petal Cream once or twice daily for four to six weeks. After that switch to the Orange Blossom Cream for the same length of time. Resume the Rose Cream and continue cycling the treatment in this way for as long as required.

To enhance the skin's ability to retain moisture, apply the cream immediately after taking a bath or shower when it is still damp. Otherwise, put some spring water in a cosmetic bottle with fine mist spray and spritz your skin.

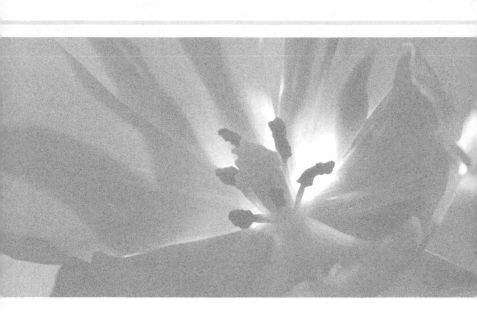

CHAPTER FOUR

Temple of the Mind

*T*here is a unique sort of relaxation and pleasure that comes from having our heads touched. Who doesn't love to go to the salon and have their hair and scalp rubbed and scrubbed by someone else, or to have a lover stroke their hair? By using certain treatments, we can bring these feelings about for ourselves. We can also treat the rest of our bodies this way, without ever moving past our head and neck.

Just like the palms of our hands and bottoms of our feet, the head is a map of nerve endings that lead directly to all our organs. Through reflexology scalp massage, depending upon where and how we touch, we can stimulate different systems throughout our beings. We can balance the *entire* body this way.

Working with the head and neck is also a way of treating the mind and spirit, because our higher chakras, the energy centers that govern our spirituality, are located here. Incorporating certain essential oils in the process can help to invigorate or calm us in the process.

Cleansing the hair and scalp also plays a role in the concept of healing the body through the crown. In certain traditions, like the Hindu chakra system, which dates back thousands of years, it is believed that positive healing energy enters the body through the head, and so it is important to have a cleared passageway through the scalp.

There are amazing benefits to head and neck treatments like scalp massages with essential oils, special neck massages, refreshing and balancing hair rinses, clay conditioners, and neck creams.

HEAD OF THE CLASS

The head is considered to be sacred in many cultures, and the hair, a symbol of power and beauty. Remember the instant weakness experienced by Samson in the Old Testament when Delilah cut his long locks? Some religions require their followers to wear head coverings, especially when in a state of prayer. Think of the yarmulkes religious Jews wear. Kings and queens wore jewels in their crowns that were meant to ward off the evil intentions of rival rulers. And throughout Asia, casually tapping someone on the head is considered to be a great offense.

Our creativity and expression are centered in this area. The crown chakra, which connects us to the divine, is our source of inspiration; the third eye chakra connects us to our inner vision; and the throat chakra, in the neck, is our center for creative expression. If you're stuck creatively, give yourself a head and neck treatment.

Chrysanthemum Eye Pillow

FROM AROGYA HOLISTIC HEALING, WESTPORT, CONNECTICUT

The Arogya Spa is holistic in that it combines traditional Chinese herbal therapies with healing modalities from all over Asia. The spa is designed in the Zen tradition—simple and peaceful.

Chrysanthemum flowers provide chi (energy) to the liver, which in Chinese medicine is connected to the eyes. This pillow can improve vision, or at least decrease puffiness in the eye area.

Dried chrysanthemum petals are available at most herbal shops and organic markets.

4 ounces dried chrysanthemum petals
1 small (3" x 8") cloth eye pillowcase

Stuff the petals into the eye pillowcase. While lying down, gently cover your eyes with the pillow for twenty minutes per day. You can also slip the eye pillow into your regular pillowcase; the aroma will help produce a more restful sleep. Drinking a cup of chrysanthemum tea will also help.

Formula for Dry Lips

**FROM STYLIST MARA SCHIAVETTI AT THE ARTE SALON,
NEW YORK, NEW YORK**

Mara Schiavetti's client list includes Nicole Kidman and Liv Tyler. Her hair and makeup styling career includes editorial work for Vogue, Glamour, *and* Marie Claire.

Here she shares with us her recipe for lip balm that she uses on location

Cat Got Your Tongue?

If you're looking for the right words to say but can't find them, massage a combination of jojoba oil and two to four drops of the following essential oils into your neck.

- For words of love, use rose oil.
- To be more creative, use jasmine oil.
- To temper and calm angry thoughts, try chamomile.
- To find words that will rouse people to action, peppermint is the oil of choice.

and in the salon. If you don't feel up to making the treatments, they can be purchased from her own company, mixdflava.com.

¼ ounce refined beeswax

2 ounces refined shea butter

1 ounce almond oil

3 drops rose or 5 drops lavender essential oil

For men, add 4 drops vanilla or 6 drops peppermint essential oil

Heat the beeswax in the top of a double boiler. Add shea butter and almond oil. When everything is melted, turn off heat and add essential oils. Pour into container and refrigerate for two hours. Take out and let stand for one hour before using.

THE NECK

In addition to housing the throat chakra, the neck is important because it is a reflex point for the reproductive system. Reproductive and hormonal problems may manifest themselves in neck aches. The reproductive system can be treated through reflex points on the neck.

At the back of the neck, we have points by which we communicate with higher realms of being. You know the sense you sometimes have that someone you know is in the room, or that the spirit of someone you loved, who passed on, is hover-

QUICKIE:
Neck Compress for Sore Throat

Feel a sore throat coming on? This can help nip it in the bud.

2–3 egg whites, beaten
2–4 drops of lavender, tea tree, or rose essential oil

Cleanse your face—and don't use moisturizer. Mix the egg whites and essential oil. Pat the mixture onto your face and neck. Massage upwards from breast to chin with sweeping motions. Let set for twenty minutes. Remove with warm water.

ing near you? You pick up on their presence from those points in the neck.

GOOD HAIR DAYS

Many of us perform a daily hair/scalp treatment: shampooing. That experience can be expanded into a healing spa treatment in a couple of ways. You can get a good, natural brush with large bristles that can invigorate your scalp while there's still shampoo or conditioner in it. Pull gently through your hair to avoid breaking the strands. You can also achieve scalp invigoration with a strong large-toothed comb. You can also add essential oils to your shampoo. In India, women put rose, sandalwood, or jasmine oil in their hair every day—just a few drops.

The idea of adding oil to hair seems foreign to many in the American culture. But just a few tiny drops will not make your hair greasy, and it will provide aromatherapy and other benefits. (I add essential oils to my unscented laundry detergent, too.)

Here are some guidelines for choosing essential oils to add to your shampoo or conditioner:

· Rosemary stimulates hair growth.
· Swiss pine halts hair loss.
· Cedarwood strengthens the hair and cleanses the scalp.
· Lemon adds shine to hair.
· Lavender thickens hair.

QUICKIE:
No More Dirty Hair

Before you get off a plane following a long flight, take a look in the bathroom mirror to see whether your hair looks dirty. Here's a quick solution if it does. And it's a great jet lag pick-me-up!

Cover your shoulders, and then sprinkle a light dusting of baby powder onto hair roots. Then towel the excess powder out of the hair. Comb or brush as usual. The powder will absorb the natural oils and rejuvenate the hair.

- Eucalyptus fights dandruff.
- Cyprus clears away grease.
- Chamomile lightens the hair color.

Sheila's Spa Scalp Treatment

FROM THE OAKS AT OJAI,

OJAI, CALIFORNIA

This treatment nourishes and strengthens the hair and revitalizes hair that has been exposed to environmental toxins. Peppermint stimulates the scalp for increased blood flow.

½ cup olive oil

2 tablespoons fresh ground lavender

2 tablespoons dried peppermint

Warm all the ingredients in small saucepan (do not boil). Massage into scalp over damp hair. Cover hair with shower cap to keep heat in. Sit in the sun, if possible, for twenty to twenty-five minutes. Shampoo and rinse hair. To be repeated once a month.

Refreshed, from the Neck Up

Want to quickly refresh your mind and spirit by way of your head and neck? At the Mandara Spa in Bali, they achieve this with towels soaked in cucumber juice and peppermint. They offer them to you as a quick energizer. You can wrap them around your head and neck, or just blot your face. It's wonderfully refreshing, and easy to do at home.

Crème Bath for Hair—with Massage

FROM THE OBEROI, LOMBOK, WEST LOMBOK, INDONESIA

This spa overlooks the Gili Islands, which are renowned for their colorful coral and fish. The beach setting is majestic, and the spa treatments are based on beauty and healing secrets passed down from generations of local village women, as well as the best of what the West has to offer.

Hair crème or conditioner
½ to 1 whole avocado, mashed, for dry hair
Aloe vera gel (for normal or oily hair)

Add avocado or aloe vera to conditioner. Apply cream onto hair and massage into scalp for a few minutes. Comb through hair and leave on for thirty minutes. Shampoo as usual.

Treatment for Dry, Brittle Hair

FROM STYLIST MARA SCHIAVETTI AT THE ARTE SALON, NEW YORK, NEW YORK

FOR DARK HAIR:

- 3 ounces shea butter
- 1 ounce jojoba oil
- 5 drops rosemary oil
- 3 drops lavender oil

FOR LIGHT HAIR

- 3 ounces shea butter
- 1 ounce jojoba oil
- 5 drops chamomile oil
- 3 drops lemon oil

Melt shea butter in the top of a double boiler with jojoba oil. Turn off heat and add essential oils. Pour into container and refrigerate for two hours. Take out and let stand for one hour before using. Wash hair with shampoo and condition. After towel-drying, apply mixture to the ends and mid lengths of your hair. Comb or finger through from scalp to ends. Don't put too much on the scalp, as that would give you an oily look.

For an intense treatment once a week or month, apply half the recipe

QUICKIE

John Stafanick at the Noelle Spa for Beauty and Wellness in Stamford, Connecticut, shares this little secret for remoisturizing a dry scalp and hair.

You can give yourself a scalp massage very easily with just a little olive oil from the cupboard. Olive oil shampoos out of hair easily and has a high moisture content.

Dip fingertips into 1 teaspoon of cold-pressed olive oil (warmed up) and massage into scalp in a circular motion for five minutes. Let set for fifteen minutes. Wash out.

Stimulating Ginger Scalp Treatment

For promoting the growth of healthy hair—a great treatment for the balding man in your life.

3 drops ginger essential oil
3 drops rosemary essential oil
1 teaspoon vegetable oil or nut oil

Mix oils together and massage into scalp for five minutes. Shampoo and rinse. Repeat at least twice a week.

to the hair and wrap in a small towel or plastic cap. Keep cap/towel on for at least half an hour and either leave the treatment in for the remainder of the day or wash it out and condition again.

For an everyday treatment, put ½ teaspoon in your palm. Rub palms together and massage the ends or dry parts of your hair.

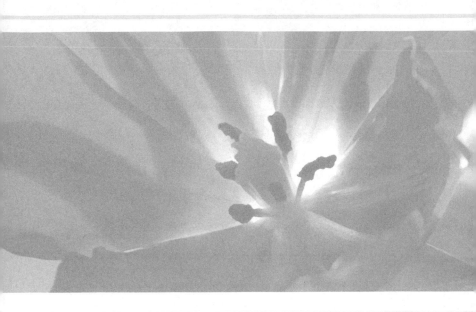

CHAPTER FIVE

Sacred Scrubs and Magical Masques

$\mathcal{M}$any people travel to exotic spas in search of a clean slate and a fresh start. This need for renewal applies not only to your thoughts and your outlook, but to your physical being as well. In fact, the two go hand in hand; in order to have a clear perspective, you need to have good physical health, and fresh, healthy skin is a very important component of that.

Fresh, younger skin is quite easy to find. It's right under the thin layer of dried, dead, toxic skin cells at the surface. Our bodies are constantly producing new cells that want to come to the surface, and we need to regularly peel away the old layers to make way for the new. To do this, we need body scrubs, with their exfoliating and detoxifying benefits.

Removing dead layers of skin opens the door for toxins and fat to exit our bodies. Scrubs can help you to lose weight, and they also allow your body to be more receptive to the nutrients in herbal baths, as well as masques.

Once we've cleared away the old skin to make room for the new, we need to welcome it gently like a baby with nourishing masques. Masques are also often referred to as wraps when they're applied before wrapping the body tightly in many layers. They can be made with rich emollients like avocado and coconut, cooling ingredients like aloe vera and cucumber, or highly nutritive elements like seaweed, herbs, or essences. Masques are a nice way to condition fresh skin, and it's a lovely way to treat your entire body to some healing agents, once your skin is better prepared for absorption. In addition to scrubs, you'll find some recipes for masques in this chapter. Of course, you don't always need to follow a scrub with a masque; but be sure to apply some oil or lotion to keep your new skin hydrated and healthy.

CLEARING THE WAY

Body scrubs are essential to maintaining overall health. Our skin is the largest organ we have. It needs to breathe, not only for itself but for the rest of the body. The skin is a permeable membrane; toxins from our internal organs need to be discharged through the skin, and beneficial nutrients need to be absorbed through it to maintain balance and health. Regularly clearing the pores of dirt and dead skin cells facilitates the release of toxins and the absorption of any healing nutrients you apply. Also, stimulating the skin with a grainy scrub promotes good circulation, another boost to toxin elimination.

"A healthy glow" is a very accurate image. There is a certain radiance that comes from going beyond superficial cleansing to a much deeper purity, a purity that detoxifying and nurturing scrubs can help us to achieve.

Exfoliating Body Scrub

FROM HOSTERIA LAS QUINTAS ECO SPA, CUERNAVACA, MEXICO

It is fitting to come to a place known as the "City of Eternal Spring" to experience the renewal of the body, mind, and spirit. Nestled in a lush valley and hidden in a "walled estate," you'll be in the midst of 100,000 square feet of lush garden, with a wide variety of exotic flowers and trees. The concept of the spa is to embrace the "whole man" concept for renewal of body and soul.

This scrub is excellent for sensitive skin and problem skin. If you suffer from psoriasis or dry, scaly skin, you'll find this recipe especially soothing and healing.

1 cup oatmeal
1 handful rose petals
½ cup honey
½ cup sea salt
1 tablespoon warm milk
Essential oil of your choice

Blend oatmeal, rose petals, honey, and sea salt into a small bowl. Add warm milk with a few drops of your favorite essential oil.

Using an exfoliating bath mitt, gently massage your body until all of the areas are covered with the mixture.

Draw a warm bath blended with bath salts and oils and soak

in the tub for twenty minutes, allowing the mixture on the body to dissolve into the tub. Rinse off completely and apply moisturizing lotion.

Mud Scrub

FROM THE PALMS AT PALM SPRINGS, PALM SPRINGS, CALIFORNIA

If you want to get fit, the staff at the Palms is committed to helping you achieve your goals. Pilates, yoga, weight-training, hiking, in-line skating— your options are numerous.

The following recipe is great for aching muscles or a general energizing detox.

2 tablespoons mud or volcanic clay (which you can get from a health
    food store or order from watermagic.com)
2 tablespoons sea salt
2 teaspoons water

Mix the ingredients together to make a slightly gummy paste. Coat the entire body, and feel the tingling as it dries. When all the moisture has left the mud, scrub it off the skin with your hands, a skin brush, a dry washcloth, or a dry loofah sponge. Your "old" skin will come off with the mud, to make way for your "new" skin. Shower. Treat your skin to a self-massage with a combination of massage oil and essential oils of your choice.

GARDEN OF VARIETY

Scrubs can be crafted for a wide variety of effects. Some are very soothing and luxurious, while others are designed for skin polishing or diminishing cellulite and wrinkles.

Gentler scrubs, for sensitive skin types or frequent use, are geared toward feeding nutrients to the body through the skin. We must be truly mindful of what we put on our skin, because it is like a sponge. Just think of all the medications now available in patch form, from nicotine for people trying to quit smoking, to nitroglycerin for those in danger of heart attacks. Why not "medicate" our bodies with healthy doses of naturally healing ingredients like essential oils, through the skin, using nutritious scrubs?

There are scrubs, like the Boreh I had at the Ritz Carlton in Bali (see page 94), which are harsher and more focused on deep-tissue detoxification. The experience during such treatments might not be the kind of bliss you have in mind when you think of visiting one of the world's most luxurious spas. They entail abrasion, and sharp hot and cold sensations. Without a doubt, afterward you emerge with a new lease on life, healthier and more vibrant that you can ever remember feeling.

The following scrubs are from famous spas and designed for various effects. What they all have in common is their exfoliating, detoxifying preparation of the skin for healthful absorption . . . and radiance. I invite you to experiment with them, and see just how rejuvenated they make you look and feel.

Salt Radiance

FROM THE DATAI, KEDAH DARUL AMAN, MALAYSIA

Imagine yourself tucked away in the midst of an ancient rain forest, totally enveloped in the mysteries of nature. A footpath through the jungle will take you to a private beach on the Andaman Sea. Here at the Datai your spa experience will nurture all your senses and put you in harmony with your inner universe.

This exfoliating scrub with sea salt and essential oils will bring forth youthful, healthy-looking skin.

1 cup sea salt

6 tablespoons vegetable oil

8 drops lavender essential oil

8 drops vetiver essential oil

8 drops ylang-ylang essential oil

Blend all ingredients.

Standing in the shower stall, massage salt and oil blend vigorously over entire body for three to five minutes, using a natural sea sponge, loofah, or washcloth.

Rinse off with cool water for energizing or hot water for relaxing.

Apply moisturizer liberally after drying off.

Rice Pure Indulgence

FROM RAJVILAS, JAIPUR, INDIA

This magnificent spa offers a natural approach that encompasses the traditional Indian Ayurvedic principles and the ancient art of aromatherapy to bring guests through the ritual of self-purification. This treatment offers three steps to rejuvenation—a scrub, a wrap, and a shower. It rehydrates, soothes, and cleanses the skin and is much easier to do if you have a partner.

Step 1: The Scrub

7 tablespoons rice flour

1 cup buttermilk (warmed)

6" x 6" muslin cloth

Put the rice flour into the muslin cloth. Tie it at the top to make a poultice. Dip the poultice into the buttermilk till soaked. Remove poultice from buttermilk and rub all over the body— except for the palms of your hands, the soles of your feet, and your face! As you move to new areas, add buttermilk to the portion of the body you are scrubbing.

Step 2: The Wrap

1 cup honey (kept warm)

Juice of two lemons

8 tablespoons rice flour

Warm water (to reduce viscosity as desired)

1 cup warm buttermilk (for very dry skin)

Large plastic sheet

Blend ingredients and lie down on the plastic sheet.

This is where a partner will help. Ask your partner to apply the honey mixture in a thick and even layer all over your body (except on the face). The partner should wrap the plastic sheet around your body and cover you with blankets to retain the heat. Relax and stay wrapped for twenty minutes.

Step 3: The Shower

Take a lukewarm shower without using any soap and apply the moisturizer of your choice after you have been out of the shower for an hour.

Bali Coffee Scrub

FROM LE MERIDIEN, TANAH LOT, BALI

The hotel and spa are located on one of Bali's most sacred sites and there is a spiritual aura of peace and sacredness that pervades the grounds. The hotel and spa are located at the ocean's edge in full view of Bali's majestic sunsets over the Tanah Lot temple. Staying at Le Meridien was like entering a very sheltered, sacred world.

Bali provides a backdrop of fairy-tale natural beauty and radiates with strong spiritual devotion. The graceful charm of Balinese hospitality combined with luxurious accommodations will embrace you and set in motion your experience of total spiritual renewal.

Bali Coffee Scrub is an intoxicatingly aromatic experience that will leave the skin smooth and polished to perfection. What do coffee and carrots have in common? Coffee will smooth and refine your skin, and at the same time elevate your mood. The mashed carrots will condition your skin and subdue the harshness of the coffee beans. This was not my idea of fun. This scrub is harsh and somewhat abrasive, but as I was quite aware of the detoxifying and purifying properties of coffee, I was willing to try it. The results are great! Just apply a liberal amount of moisturizer afterwards.

  1 cup finely ground coffee beans
  3 tablespoons cosmetic clay or dried mud
  1 cup mashed grated raw carrots
  1 teaspoon gelatin

Crush coffee beans finely and mix with cosmetic clay. Add a little water. Rub over body, taking your time to give the skin a good exfoliation. For extra exfoliation, use a natural loofah. Remove excess scrub with a damp cloth.

Mix the carrot with the gelatin and apply to entire body, gently massaging onto the skin.

Rinse off and enjoy the day!

Refreshing and stimulating, this treatment is aimed at rejuvenating the skin and arousing the senses.

The Icing on the Cake

No matter what kind of scrub you choose, it is important to moisturize your skin at the end of the process. You can use your favorite lotion or massage oil, and I recommend mixing in some essential oils.

THE LUXURIOUS LULUR

On my last visit to the region, I was treated to a Lulur at the Oberoi on the majestic Indonesian island of Lombok. What made it extra special was that I was able to experience it with my then-boyfriend, Charlie. There's an especially sensual quality to the Lulur, because of its gentleness and the fragrant flowers and oils included in the three-step process. It's no wonder it plays a role in preparing couples for marriage. Knowing this about the Lulur adds a certain romance. While it's absolutely wonderful to experience a Lulur alone, it can be very special to share it with your partner.

At the Oberoi, Charlie and I were sent to a changing room together where we had been instructed to dress in disposable rice panties and a sarong. We then lay on side-by-side massage tables. First, our entire bodies were scrubbed with a mildly abrasive combination of massage oil, rice powder, sandalwood oil, and bright yellow turmeric. Any heat generated by the spicy scrub was then cooled by the application of fresh yogurt everywhere. We relaxed for a few minutes, coated with this delicious skin salve, before we were led to wash off at an outdoor shower overlooking endless Lombok greenery and the ocean. I already felt refreshed, and there were still two more parts to the treatment! Next, Charlie and I were guided to a big marble bathtub for two, which was brimming with warm water and fantastically fragrant flowers. While we soaked, we were served stimulating ginger tea. Who knew detoxification could be so luxurious? Finally, we were taken back to the massage tables for a full-body massage with healing essential oils.

After our two hours of total bliss, we were ready to return to our oceanfront villa for a romantic evening together.

This treatment is messy, but well worth the cleanup. I recommend you cover your treatment area with old sheets or towels.

Luxurious Lulur

FROM THE OBEROI, LOMBOK, WEST LOMBOK, INDONESIA

2 teaspoons finely ground rice powder

2 teaspoons turmeric

1 teaspoon sandalwood essential oil

Your favorite massage oil

2 cups fresh yogurt (plain)

3 drops jasmine essential oil

As many fragrant flowers as you can gather

Combine the rice powder, turmeric, and sandalwood oil. Cover your skin with massage oil, then apply the turmeric mixture and let it dry for a few minutes before scrubbing it off.

Coat the skin with yogurt, and feel it moisturizing. Relax for a few minutes. Shower. Then draw a hot bath and fill it with the flowers and jasmine oil. It helps to drink tea or hot lemon water while you're soaking.

Finally, give yourself an all-over self-massage with massage oil and any essential oils whose fragrances you love. (Go to your local health food store to explore essential oils, and discover which ones invigorate or calm your senses. For example, laven-

Maybe you can't fly to Indonesia every time you want to experience a Lulur or other treatment—but you don't have to. You can create a certain environment within your home that can transport you to another place, while you're scrubbing and soaking and relaxing.

Lighting is a great way to transform an environment. If you have a fluorescent light on the ceiling, shut it off and bring a small, low-voltage lamp into the bathroom. Or light fragrant candles, just as many as you need to provide enough light to see.

Another visual and physiological treat can be provided by plants. You can recruit these beautiful oxygen providers from anywhere in the house for your special hour. Or buy some tall tropical plants to keep in the bathroom all the time. It will feel much more like paradise.

You can also play with sound in your special environment. Put some soft music on the stereo or find some special atmospheric music in the New Age section of your local music store. You can find recordings of environmental sounds or indigenous music that will make you forget where you are.

der calms, while peppermint awakens and stimulates. See page 32 for the beneficial properties of essential oils.)

COCONUT SCRUB

Scrubbing the skin doesn't have to be a harsh experience. There are softer, more gentle scrubs that can help exfoliate the surface, but are more geared toward softening the skin and fortifying it with nutritious moisture.

What could be more soothing to sensitive skin than cool, silky coconut? Coconut is abundant in tropical cultures, and has been used for centuries to heal and condition the skin. It is rich in emollient oils and other vitamins and nutrients. Mixed with mild abrasives, like turmeric, coconut can be used as a scrub.

Coconut-Carrot Polish

FROM THE TAJ EXOTICA, SOUTH MALE ATOLL, MALDIVES

A secluded, peaceful island resort, the Taj Exotica offers treatments in the Asian tradition and therapies that represent a global fusion of influences from Bali, Europe, Hawaii, Japan, and China. The Maldives, off the coast of India, are truly a feast for the senses.

1 grated coconut, preferably fresh
½ teaspoon turmeric powder
½ pound grated carrots
½ cup gelatin, already set

Make a mixture of the coconut and turmeric and coat the body with it. Once it is dry, gently scrub this paste off the body, using a moist cloth. Combine the carrots and gelatin and coat the skin for a cooling, moisturizing treat to further soothe the skin. Rinse under a warm shower.

DEEP DETOX: THE BOREH BODY SCRUB

I can't think of any spa treatment that is more intense—or more healing for the entire body—than the Boreh body scrub, another ancient Indonesian formulation that is practiced by all the spas in that area. The Boreh has its roots in Bali. The people there have used this scrub for ages, as an antidote for colds, fever, the flu, and other infections. The Boreh can also be used periodically as a preventative measure, to keep the body clear of threatening toxins and microbes. It can even relieve jet lag and general malaise.

Because of its intensity, this scrub is not for everyone. There are some harsh, burning sensations and some chills, which are essential to deep-tissue detoxification. In fact, the benefits of a Boreh scrub are dramatic, probably ten times more detoxifying than everyday scrubs.

When I was in Bali last, I decided to try a Boreh scrub at the Ritz Carlton. I was out of balance and feeling quite out of sorts because of severe jet lag. At the Ritz Carlton, I was treated like royalty, with my own private villa looking over trees and rice paddies. I knew I was in for something special. But I didn't know it was going to feel more like medicine than like pampering.

The spices in this scrub are designed to create heat on the outside of the body, which stimulates circulation and the discharge of toxins from the internal organs. As I lay there, covered in the spicy, traditional Boreh paste, I felt like my skin was burning. At the same time, I was having internal chills, the kind that accompany a virus. It's the same experience: all of your organs are working hard to expel unwanted particles and pass them along through the circulatory system and the skin.

When it was over, though, I felt like a new woman. I had incredible energy and alertness and was in a wonderful mood. I felt as if I could achieve anything. My body felt refreshed and relaxed, from the inside out, and my jet lag had mirac-

QUICKIE:
Low-Maintenance Scrubs in a Pinch

Let's face it: you don't always have time for an involved scrub treatment with several steps and ingredients. But that doesn't mean you can't fit the healing and beautifying benefits of a body scrub into your routine. There are much quicker recipes, which you can enjoy on even your busiest days.

Salt and Oil scrub: As simple as it sounds. Simply slather on your favorite vegetable oil and then scrub your body with a handful of sea salt. Rinse in the shower, and then moisturize with your favorite lotion.

Aloe Vera and Lavender Oil Scrub: This is an especially gentle scrub because there are no abrasives involved. Simply mix fresh aloe vera gel from the health food store (or from a plant frond) with a few drops of lavender oil. Cover your body with the mixture and let it dry. Then brush the dried aloe off with your hands or a dry cloth. While the aloe softens and exfoliates your skin, the lavender balances your mind. Notice how renewed you feel.

ulously disappeared. Back to my best self, I could now begin my vacation.

Boreh

FROM THE RITZ CARLTON JALAN KARANG MAS SEJATERA,

JIMBARAN, BALI, INDONESIA

Perched on a bluff overlooking the Indian Ocean, this magnificent hotel and spa offers treatments based on Balinese and Javanese beauty rituals and well-being treatments handed down through generations.

2 teaspoons ground black pepper

2 teaspoons whole cloves

4 teaspoons sandalwood

2 teaspoons ground ginger

1 teaspoon cinnamon

1 teaspoon coriander seeds

2 teaspoons finely ground rice powder

1 teaspoon turmeric

1 teaspoon nutmeg

1 teaspoon massage oil

4 grated carrots

Make a paste of all these ingredients, except the grated carrots. For more sensitive skin, use more rice powder, and dilute with more massage oil and water. Coat the skin with the paste, and then cover the body with sheets and blankets to promote heating and detoxification. Remain still for about twenty minutes, enduring the burning and chilling sensations. Breathe. Focus on positive thoughts. Then rub the dried paste off the skin vigorously. Finally, cool and moisturize the skin by coating it with cooling carrots for five minutes or so. Then shower and apply additional massage oil, with your favorite essential oil added to it, to the skin.

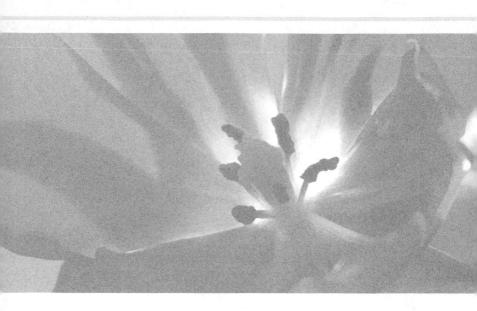

CHAPTER SIX

Bathing the Spirit

athing has wonderful medicinal and spiritual values. Of all the spa treatments that have been passed down from ancient cultures, the bath is the easiest to achieve, and one of the most effective.

Bathing has been significant not only in great healing traditions throughout the ages, but in religious and mystical ceremonies in ancient Egypt, Rome, and Greece, and all major religions. Hot springs throughout Asia have been used for centuries for both spiritual cleansing and medicinal treatments.

More than a cleansing and healing opportunity, bathing gives us a chance to connect to our inner selves, to our higher selves, and to a higher power.

We are all familiar with the comforting, womblike experience of soaking in warm water. Add certain essential oils, salts, or flowers, and the experience becomes completely transporting.

You can take yourself to other places within yourself and within your imagination. The bath transforms your state of mind, creating ideal conditions for meditation and creative visualization. In the bath, we can allow our spirits to soar. And when our spirits are free, we are free—to heal, to be ourselves, to create, to prepare to follow our dreams without limitations.

While you're off on your mental journey, the healing ingredients you use in the tub will be absorbed by your skin to act on your entire system. The cleansing and healing benefits help to put us in good physical health, which naturally promotes good emotional and spiritual health.

HEALING FROM THE OUTSIDE IN

The physical benefits behind baths have been well documented throughout history. At one time, bathing was the number-one doctor-prescribed remedy for virtually every ailment under the sun. At seaside spas, patients were instructed to have baths, or "take the waters," often with salt, herbs, or essential oils mixed in.

Bathing plays a key role in detoxification, flushing unwanted elements from our bodies, especially when we incorporate sea salts and other additives with drawing properties. But bathing can also play a role in feeding and nurturing the body. Amazingly, the substances we bathe in can affect not just our skin, but our entire bodies.

The skin is the largest organ of the body, and a direct conduit between the outside and our internal organs. What we put on it quickly enters our bloodstream and is then circulated throughout the body. For instance, if you soak in a bath treated with lavender, and then take a hair sample a half hour later, there will be traces of lavender in your hair.

Refer to the chart on essential oils and their healing properties on page 32 to help you select oils to bathe in. Or use the bath recipes provided here from spas around the world.

BATHTUB BLISS

There's a certain luxury associated with baths—think of the decadent bubble bath—that relaxed, pampered feeling is part of what makes baths so good for you: you're treating yourself to some time out for something that feels good and is good for you, while building your self-esteem.

QUICKIE:
Lavender Shower Wash

Lavender has a healing power that is extremely diverse and has been used in ancient cultures for healing and cleansing. The botanical name *Lavendula* comes from the Latin *lavare*, meaning "to wash." The pure, clean fragrance conjures up images of innocence—something untouched, which washes away impurities of body and mind. It is also known to have a stimulating effect on the skin and is particularly good for dry skin.

Add fifteen drops of lavender essential oil to liquid soap. Massage Lavender Body Wash over entire body. Remove with a wet washcloth or sponge.

Let's not forget the sensual aspects. There are certain bath oils that can have an aphrodisiac effect. Cleopatra is said to have implemented aromatic bathing as a seduction ritual, sweetening the scent of her skin with fragrances designed specifically to lure Marc Antony. There are sensual baths for lovers, too. Some of the most connected together time with your lover can be in a warm, fragrant bath.

Bathing in the company of others isn't new; in fact, bathing wasn't always a solo affair. In the past, bathing was a public, social endeavor. As early as medieval times, the well-to-do in Europe would spend time together in communal baths, gossiping, drinking, and snacking. Throughout Europe, Russia, Japan, and Turkey, bathhouses were famous retreats where people would bathe together, sip tea, and generally hang out. It actually happens today, too, in Jacuzzis and whirlpools at ski resorts and spas, although today we have the benefit of swimsuits to cover us up, if we want to.

JUMP IN

It's time to make some time for yourself, and get into a luxurious tubful of fragrant waters. Remember—you are not here in this world to merely survive and endure the struggles of everyday life. You deserve time to discover yourself and enjoy yourself.

Make sure you give yourself ample time to relax into the experience, and to gently come out of it when you're done. Remember that this is your time for nurturing and self-indulgence—and that it's necessary in order for you to have the energy to take care of all the other people in your life. Select a spa recipe that fits your mood or your condition. Then send the kids on a play date, shut off the phone, put on some lovely music, light some candles, and let your body and mind be gently lulled to a different consciousness by the warm water and the soothing flowers or oils you choose. Create an atmosphere of peacefulness and harmony. Allow your mind to truly relax and to float

QUICKIE:
Travel to the Tropics with Your Partner on a Cold Winter's Night

Fill a tub with water and three or more cups of flower blossoms (the more the better). Add ten to twelve drops of the essential oil of choice—rose, jasmine, and orange blossom are some sensual ones. You can even use a combination.

Flower petals can be obtained from your local florist at the end of the day when they discard flowers that are not fit for market. Usually, flowers from flower shops are sprayed with pesticides. To remove the pesticides, add two tablespoons of Clorox to a bowl full of water or use a commercial product available in a health food store and soak blossoms for a minute or two.

away to the most blissful spot you can imagine in all the world. Stop the chatter, the judgments, the planning for tomorrow. Let your seriousness melt away and be replaced with joy and gaiety. Before you know it, you'll wonder where all your stress has gone, and your spirit will feel alive again.

Energizing Rose Hip Oil Treatment with Body Brush

FROM THE ROSEWATER SPA OF OAKVILLE, OAKVILLE, ONTARIO, CANADA

The mission of the Rosewater Spa is to inspire serenity. The spa is dedicated to offering clients the enjoyment of good health in restful surroundings through therapeutic massage and restorative body and skin treatments.

Step 1: Body Brushing

Perhaps one of the simplest and most underestimated therapies, dry skin body brushing has been found to play an important part in stimulating vital energy flow. Use the body brush (a natural-fiber brush with a wooden handle, found at health food stores) to massage every part of your body. Make rotary motions, then finish with long strokes upwards toward your heart. Begin with the soles of your feet, move up your legs, and don't forget your hands, arms, back (a brush with a long handle will help you to do this alone), abdomen, chest, neck, and face.

Brush for five to ten minutes, until your skin is glowing.

Step 2: The Bath

Solstice Sunburst Tub Tea (available at many health food stores; or, to make your own tea, combine orange peels, yellow rose petals, and 8 to 12 drops sweet orange essential oil)

This bath helps to eliminate toxin buildup, relaxes muscles and tissues, and opens pores to allow better penetration of oils.

Put into a sock (no holes, please) three rounded tablespoons of Tub Tea, or your own mixture of orange peels, flower petals, and sweet orange essential oil. The color yellow—the color of sunshine—is important here. Dunk the sock into the bathwater as a tea bag for the tub, and let it steep. Lower yourself into the tub. Relax and enjoy. Imagine the invigorating energy of the sun revitalizing you.

Just What the Doctor Ordered

We all know what baths can do for our state of mind. But did you know they can improve your heart rate, increase your oxygen consumption, and boost your cardiac efficiency? That's what a 1994 study in Japan revealed. Patients who regularly took fifteen-minute baths enjoyed all these benefits, the researchers believe, because of the way warm water dilates arteries and veins and increases blood flow from the heart and lungs. This is not to mention all the detoxifying and cleansing benefits. Is there anything a bath can't do for you?

Step 3: Rose Hip Oil Treatment

Rose hip oil

Body lotion or a carrier oil, like jojoba, almond, or sesame

After your bath, massage a mixture of rose hip oil and either lotion or a carrier oil into the skin. You need very little—only about twelve drops. Rose hip oil contains ten to one hundred times more vitamin C than any other food, making this oil a most powerful antioxidant and incredibly beneficial to your skin.

Rose hip oil also contains calcium, iron, and phosphorus, vitamins B_1, B_2, A, E, K, P, and niacin. It strengthens capillary walls, rejuvenates growth of healthy tissue, including scar tissue, hydrates skin tissues, repairs signs of premature aging, and nourishes the scalp and hair—especially chemically treated hair.

Step 4: Rose Hip Oil Misting

Rose hip oil

Water

Mix twelve drops of rose hip oil with two ounces of water in a spray bottle, and mist your whole body. This water is cleansing and mildly astringent. It will hydrate and refresh your skin.

QUICKIE:
Fennel Bath

For a calm mind and peaceful spirit.

5 or more fennel stalks

Boil five or more fennel stalks. Strain the water and add to bathwater.

As you sit in the bath, concentrate on your breathing to focus your mind. This will allow the calming effects of the fennel to relax you more quickly.

Kneipp Hydrotherapy Immune Builder

FROM THE STERLING INSTITUTE SPA, SANTA FE, NEW MEXICO

*The philosophy of the Sterling Institute is "good health through healthy living."
The spa is committed to educating its clients and believes that if we supply the
body with what it needs, it can balance itself.*

*This shower is a great body rejuvenator. It strengthens the immune sys-
tem by increasing circulation and keeping the autonomic nervous system
responsive. It's especially good in the morning as a substitute for coffee or
anytime your system needs a boost. If you are prone to colds, make this a
weekly ritual. The rosemary essential oil is also an antidote for morning
grouchiness.*

Dry body brush
Kneipp Rosemary Shower Gel (or add 12 drops rosemary essential oil
    to your bath gel)
1 lemon, cut in half

Brush your dry skin for at least five minutes.

Shower with Rosemary Shower Gel, and end your shower
with a cold-water rinse.

Complete your treatment by rubbing half of the lemon all
over your skin for added rejuvenation. Squeeze the juice of the
other half of the lemon into a glass of water and drink up. This
will help your liver to function more efficiently.

WELCOME TO YOUR HOME SPA

Half the experience at any spa comes from the environment. When you travel to the spas of Asia or the Caribbean, part of the experience is outdoors, with lots of lush plants everywhere. In Europe and the United States, many of the spas are beautifully designed and appointed, with beautifully subtle lighting. If you can't get to a spa, then change the atmosphere where you are about to do your spa treatment. Here's how to make your bathroom feel like a different, more exotic place:

- Light many candles for softer illumination. Choose some that are scented with essential oils, for the aromatherapy benefits.
- Bring some plants and/or flowers into the room, for aromatherapy and more oxygen. An excellent plant for creating good air is the golden pathos.
- Use some luxurious soaps, naturally scented with essential oils.
- Add natural sea sponges for a lovely touch; they are gently exfoliating.
- Use a bath pillow—this will make a long bath a more comfortable option.
- Buy some special thick, long towels that are exclusively for your spa experiences.
- Pick up a luxurious robe, slippers, and perhaps a hair clip and towel.

QUICKIE:
Oatmeal Sponge for Dry, Itchy, Scaly Skin

Oatmeal is a gentle water softener and has a healing and particularly soothing effect on irritated skin.

Place a cupful of oatmeal in a cheesecloth bag and secure it. Use as a sponge when you shower or take a bath. You may also add a few drops of your favorite essential oil to honey or liquid soap inside the sponge and submerge it in bathwater.

The sponge will last through three to five baths.

- Choose some soothing music and play it softly.
- Make sure that everyone else in the house knows this is your time, and you are not to be disturbed! Even if it means putting a Do Not Disturb sign on the door.

California Citrus Bath

FROM THE OAKS AT OJAI SPA, OJAI, CALIFORNIA

The Oaks at Ojai is truly a stress-free environment. This spa offers healthy spa cooking, guided hikes, yoga, and a wide array of treatments, including hot river rock massages, body scrubs, hypnotherapy, reflexology, aromatherapy wraps, and more.

This invigorating bath will create an overall feeling of well-being and leave you feeling refreshed. The lime is for stimulation, lemon to treat lethargy, and orange to reduce depression and anxiety. Dried parsley is also for stimulation and the oatmeal is to soften the water.

¼ cup grated lime peel

¼ cup grated lemon peel

4 cups grated orange peel

1 tablespoon dried parsley

2 tablespoons oatmeal

Mix ingredients and add to bathwater.

"Bath" on the Run: Getting More Out of Your Shower

Most days, we don't have time for a long, luxurious bath. In fact, many of us barely have time to shower. But we can turn our precious few showering minutes into a spa experience that will help to make the rest of the day go more smoothly.

- Put a few drops of an essential oil that you like to use for aromatherapy into the bottom of the tub and close the drain as if you are going to take a bath. Then, run the shower. You'll benefit from the oils in two ways: you'll breathe them in, and they'll be absorbed through your feet. I use eucalyptus oil for my eighty-year-old mother when she can't breathe. It has saved us many trips to the emergency room.
- Place some sea salts in the shower, too, for detoxification through your feet and for converting negative energy to positive.
- Do a quickie scrub before jumping in, by rubbing your skin with jojoba or even vegetable oil and sea salt.
- As you stand under the water, envision white light showering through your body and cleansing you at every level—physical, emotional, and spiritual—and removing all your tensions.
- Visualize achieving your goals for the day—or the year, or your life—as your mind relaxes and you breathe in the scents of whatever oil you have chosen.

The Benefits of Chocolate
(Courtesy of the Hershey Spa)

- Today we know that contrary to common belief, chocolate is packed with nutrients and antioxidants that are thought to reduce the risk of cancer.
- Chocolate also contains theobromine, which is related to caffeine and phenylethylanine, an antidepressant that exists naturally in the human brain.
- Cocoa is conceivably a treasure chest of compounds which potentially have beneficial effects on human health.
- There are indications that some of the 600 chemicals so far found in the cocoa bean could help protect the human immune system, fight rheumatism, and combat stress.
- Japanese experiments have also shown that cocoa extracts could help reduce excessive immune reactions, act against factors that cause rheumatism, and reduce the effects of stress. In a stress test that could have implications for commuters on crowded subway trains, rats dosed with cocoa polyphenols remained calmer than others crowded into a confined space with them.
- Harvard School of Public Health researchers, led by epidemiologist Dr. I-Min Lee, studied food questionnaires answered by nearly 8,000 male Harvard graduates and found that those who ate a "moderate" amount of candy (one to three candy bars a month) lived a year longer than those who didn't.
- A drink to our health! A rich cup of cocoa may be as good for the heart as it is for the soul. Researchers at the University of California at Davis report that the chocolatey drink can actually help stave off a stroke or heart attack by preventing blood clots from forming.

Just like aspirin, cocoa is believed to work its magic by interfering with the normal functioning of platelets, tiny blood cells that can clump together inside your arteries.

Whipped Cocoa Bath

FROM THE HERSHEY SPA, HERSHEY, PENNSYLVANIA

Nestled atop a hill overlooking the famous Hershey Gardens, this is a full-service, European-style spa. The spa incorporates indigenous ingredients of chocolate and roses into innovative treatments.

This is a signature chocolate treatment from the Hershey Spa. The milk powder softens and soothes the skin, while the lactic acid contained in the diluted powder helps exfoliate and renew the skin. Imagine sitting in a warm cup of hot chocolate. . . .

⅛ cup Hershey's unsweetened cocoa powder

⅓ cup instant nonfat dry milk powder

½ cup Whipped Cocoa Bath (a foaming product formulated exclusively for the Spa at the Hotel Hershey)

This bath is best experienced in a whirlpool tub, creating a frothy, foamy effect. If you have a regular tub, you will derive the benefits, but miss out on playing in the foam.

Add cocoa powder and milk powder to bathwater while tub is filling. Add the whipped Cocoa Bath and turn on the whirlpool.

Oceanic Ritual: The Island Spa's Tribute to the Sea

FROM THE ISLAND SPA AT THE FOUR SEASONS RESORT MALDIVES, AT
KUDA HURAA, MALDIVES

Perched at the edge of this private island spa's white sandy beach, overlooking the turquoise ocean, are five thatched-roof treatment pavilions designed for couples spa experiences. Innovative treatments from India, Thailand, Indonesia, and the Maldives are offered, incorporating ancient regional traditions with the finest natural ingredients.

- 2–3 teaspoons Zeal Oil (a signature Four Seasons blend; you can substitute with your own blend of essential oils (mandarin, grapefruit, black pepper, and basil)
- ¼ to ½ cup sea salt
- 12 drops citrus blend essential oils (orange blossom, lemon, grapefruit, lime, tangerine)
- ½–1 cup coconut milk
- 2–3 vanilla beans

Begin by massaging the energizing blend of Zeal Oil onto your body.

Follow by rubbing sea salt onto the skin to exfoliate the dead cells.

Next luxuriate in a bath to which you've added a total of twelve drops of a combination of citrus essential oils (orange blossom, lemon, grapefruit, lime, tangerine).

Add the coconut milk and whole vanilla beans or a few drops

of vanilla extract to your bath and imagine you're on your own tropical island paradise without a care in the world.

SALT BATHS

The Dead Sea is one of the world's most ancient healing sites. Cleopatra, the Queen of Sheba, and Roman gladiators all recognized Dead Sea salts for their curative powers—and their powers are many.

Dead Sea salts' unique and high concentration of minerals has the ability to alleviate dermatological problems such as psoriasis and eczema. A young girl who worked for me who had terrible itching and scaling all over her body (and was too embarrassed to date because of it), started using our Dead Sea Salts and was able to cure her condition.

Dead Sea salts have a high concentration of minerals:

- Magnesium—promotes healing
- Bromides—have a tranquilizing effect on the nervous system
- Iodine—helps balance the metabolism

QUICKIE:
Partner's Bath—Soft and Sweet (or Sweet, Sexy, and Sensual . . .)

From body treatment specialist Sandy Kiman at the Noelle Spa for Beauty and Wellness, this treatment exfoliates and moisturizes the skin and enhances the senses. It is excellent for those whose skin is too sensitive for salt scrubs. The enzymes in the sugar will exfoliate and soften the skin and the oil will lubricate and hydrate the skin. What you end up with is skin that is soft, smooth, and sexy. What a great way to begin a romantic evening at home.

1 cup sugar
¼ cup warmed oil
6 drops sexy essential oil, like rose, jasmine, ginger, or ylang-ylang
2 sponges

Mix sugar, oil, and fragrance into a body scrub. Sponge all over your partner's body.

- Calcium—calms and soothes
- Potassium—relaxes

Dead Sea salts are highly effective in relieving:

- Muscle cramps
- Joint and muscle pain
- Neck pain and back aches

Dead Sea Salt Bath

FROM THE SANCTUARY ZARA SPA, AMMAN, JORDAN

The concept of the Sanctuary Zara Spa is holistic, treating the mind, body, and spirit through a focus on relaxation and beauty treatments. The atmosphere of the spa, at the edge of the Dead Sea, is rich with ancient mystery and traditions of natural healing.

½ cup sea salt
2 tablespoons carrier oil, such as jojoba, sesame, olive, or almond

Mix the salt and oil together, and scrub them all over the body, exfoliating dead skin. Then get into tub full of water and soak. You can also rinse the scrub off in the shower, if you are short on time.

JAPANESE BATHS

In the fall of 2000, I was invited to Japan to teach classes in aromatherapy and polarity therapy. I spent two weeks in Japan, totally immersed in a culture in which the ritual of bathing plays a major role.

The Japanese bath has deep spiritual roots, originating with the ancient Shinto religion, a religion which honors nature and emphasizes purification. Originally, the bath was part of a healing and purifying ritual. The water was infused with medicinal herbs and oils. The combination of the hot water, aromatic oils and herbs, along with the intention of healing was very powerful.

The bath is still an integral part of Japanese culture. It can be found everywhere from small country inns and large hotels to communal bathhouses and hot springs in beautiful settings. In each Japanese house there is a deep tub for hot-water baths. Each person showers before entering the tub. Herbs, flowers, or leaves are added to the water. There is often a beautiful scene of nature or objects of beauty to contemplate while bathing.

Ceremony is a strong part of Japanese life. One Japanese man, a student of mine, described his feelings about the bath as a time to let down all defenses, to be infused with the spirit of the water. He further explained that the Japanese word for God is *Kami,* which is broken down into two words: *Ka,* meaning "fire," and *mi,* meaning "water." When these two elements are mixed, warm water is born. As the Japanese bathe,

QUICKIE:
Buttermilk Bath

Add a quart of buttermilk to your bathwater to moisturize and beautify the skin. The lactic acid in buttermilk acts as a gentle exfoliant to soften the skin. Buttermilk softens and soothes without a sour smell.

they feel the warm water transforming their spirit and healing the body. In this context, the bath can bring renewal and spiritual awakening.

Hot Spring Bath

FROM THE HAKONE PRINCE HOTEL, KANAGAWA, JAPAN

The open-air hot spring spa at Prince Hotel has a view of Lake Ashi, the lush surrounding forests and the magnificent Mount Fuji. This mystical setting has become a mountaintop oasis for weary travelers seeking to revitalize the body and spirit in the wonderful herb baths and steam baths featured at the spa. I came here after teaching for two straight weeks in Tokyo. Maya and her sister Hiroka initiated me into the Japanese bathing ritual. For me it was a profound mystical experience. We were the only ones in the outdoor hot mineral bath at the base of Mount Fuji on a lake on a very foggy, misty night. With mist and steam giving our naked bodies some degree of privacy we ventured out to the sandy shore of Lake Ashi and chanted.

Although not an adequate substitute for going to this spa, this is a beneficial bath nonetheless.

3 cups sea salt

3 tablespoons seaweed

QUICKIE:
Quick Detox

This is a great skin refresher before an important night out, guaranteed to make your skin glow.

1–2 cups sake (Japanese rice wine)

Add sake to bathwater and soak for fifteen to twenty minutes.

Wash and shower first. Add sea salt and seaweed to the hottest temperature water that you are comfortable in. Think peaceful thoughts while your body is being remineralized.

Note: If you are pregnant or have a heart condition or other medical problem the water should not be too hot.

Ancient Moroccan Ritual with Rhassoul Black Clay

FROM THE LAUSANNE PALACE AND SPA, LAUSANNE, SWITZERLAND

The Lausanne Palace and Spa is a place of extraordinary beauty and elegance, where history has been written by kings and world leaders. The spa's philosophy of healing and well-being incorporates the world's best therapies including Ayurveda, Bach Flower Remedies, color therapy, qi gong, and thalasotherapy.

Rhassoul is a black clay extracted from the earth south of fez Morocco. This mysterious and healing clay has played an important role in life on earth due to its virtues in storing and transferring energy, which gives it its healing power and reputation as being the most ancient healing treatment in the world.

10 drops of your favorite essential oil

Olive oil soap or any good exfoliating soap

1 cup Rhassoul (black clay) or any high-quality clay

Orange blossom water (or 12 drops orange blossom essential oil in
2 ounces water)

Begin with an essential oil steam bath to open pores. Steam up your bathroom, adding essential oils to the tub's closed drain, or take a bath in a steamed-up bathroom with your added essential oils.

Cover your face with a damp, ice-cold washcloth to protect the epidermis from the heat of the steam.

Next, exfoliate the skin with an olive oil soap. Exfoliation rids the skin of dead cells and prepares it to receive the Rhassoul clay.

Mix Rhassoul clay with warm water until it becomes a mud and apply it from head to toe. Let the wrap harden and leave on for ten to twenty minutes.

Wash off and apply an essential oil–based body oil or lotion. The oil will complete the process, promoting the smoothness of skin and tightening the pores.

End your ritual with a head-to-toe sprinkling of orange blossom water for harmonizing the self and pacifying the soul.

Please note that if you cannot find Rhassoul clay, you can substitute another high-quality clay, but keep in mind that each clay has its own unique properties.

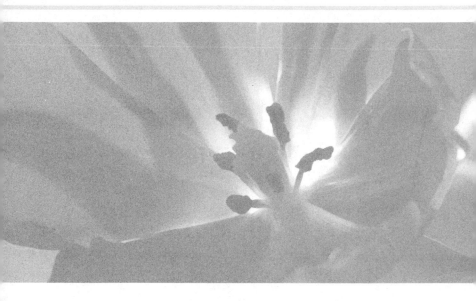

CHAPTER SEVEN

Balancing Extremities

*O*ur hands and our feet do so much for us. We work with them, eat with them, scrub dishes with them, walk on them, stand on them, and then what do *we* do for *them*?

When we treat them in a certain way, it is possible to realign and balance our entire bodies through our extremities. In the palms of our hands and on the soles or our feet are reflex points that correspond to every organ in our bodies. When we learn certain massage techniques, called reflexology, we can manipulate various body systems while also relieving tension and achieving relaxation.

Another interesting property of our hands and feet is that they have the largest pores within the entire epidermis, and so they absorb essential oils and nutrients in baths, scrubs, and masques more easily than other areas of the body. Just as with the skin covering the rest of our bodies, we first need to clear away the top layer of old cells on our hands and feet with exfoliating scrubs. Then we need to treat the fresh, absorbent young cells with care, softening them with gentle masques and lotions.

ENERGY FLOW

The flow of energy through our beings is key to the quality of our lives. Blockages manifest themselves in tension, negativity, illness, and not looking our best. The field of study called polarity examines the way energy flows through us. A simplified explanation of polarity is that positive energy enters us through the tops of our heads, and negative energy exits through our feet.

To take this further, there are energy currents called meridians that run down each side of the body. These meridians are the basis for acupuncture and some other Eastern energy-healing modalities.

Because the feet expel negative energy, it is very important to keep them clean and clear—well scrubbed and exfoliated so that no negativity gets trapped.

Positive energy, on the other hand, comes in through the top of the head and flows through our hands. We express so much with our hands. We prepare food for our loved ones with them, write with them, draw with them. We touch each other with them, and that has so much positive power. We channel much of our creative expression through our hands, so we need to keep them clean and clear.

Keeping the energy currents in the hands and feet open will have a positive effect on the rest of the body, too.

Aromatherapy Salt Glo
For Hands And Feet

FROM THE OAKS AT OJAI, OJAI, CALIFORNIA

The Oaks offers a serene, yet upbeat atmosphere. The spa places an emphasis on fitness. After you've sampled one of the sixteen daily fitness classes, it's time to enjoy an aromatic, soothing treatment.

3 tablespoons sea salt

1 cup grape seed or almond oil

8–10 drops of your favorite essential oil

Mix grape seed or almond oil and sea salt into a paste. For feet, add extra salt to increase exfoliating effect. Apply to skin and leave on for five minutes.

Remove with a warm washcloth with a few drops of essential oil on it. The salt melts with the heat of the body and the skin absorbs the minerals. The essential oil is absorbed into the bloodstream. (Lavender oil will produce a calming and detoxifying effect. Chamomile oil is excellent for the feet, too. It reduces inflammation, dryness, and itching.)

REFLEXOLOGY EXPLAINED

As with the face and the head, when we treat the hands and feet, we are treating the rest of the body through nerve endings and reflex points. There is a special healing modality associated with this, called reflexology.

Laura Norman's Foot Reflexology Chart

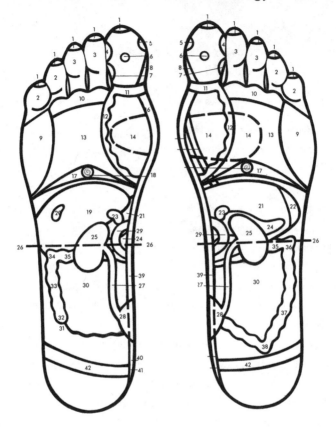

1. Brain	**13.** Chest/lung	**28.** Bladder
2. Sinuses/outer ear	**14.** Heart	**29.** Duodenum
3. Sinuses/inner ear/eye	**15.** Esophagus	**30.** Small intestine
4. Temple	**16.** Thoracic spine (T1–T12)	**31.** Appendix
5. Pineal/hypothalamus	**17.** Diaphragm	**32.** Illeocecal valve
6. Pituitary	**18.** Solar plexus	**33.** Ascending colon
7. Side of neck	**19.** Liver	**34.** Hepatic flexure
8. Cervical spine (C1–C7)	**20.** Gallbladder	**35.** Transverse colon
9. Shoulder/arm	**21.** Stomach	**36.** Splenic flexure
10. Neck/helper to eye, inner ear, eustachian tube	**22.** Spleen	**37.** Descending colon
	23. Adrenals	**38.** Sigmoid colon
	24. Pancreas	**39.** Lumbar spine (L1–L5)
11. Neck/thyroid/ parathyroid/tonsils	**25.** Kidney	**40.** Sacral spine
	26. Waistline	**41.** Coccyx
12. Bronchial/thyroid helper	**27.** Ureter tube	**42.** Sclatic nerve

The ancient art of reflexology has been practiced for at least five thousand years in India, China, and Egypt. Reflexology is a therapy that involves applying pressure to certain points, called reflex points, in the hands and feet that correspond to internal organs and systems. The benefits include improved circulation, detoxification of the physical and emotional body, relaxation, balancing of the auric field, and healing of internal organs. By treating the hands and/or feet with reflexology, you can treat the rest of the body.

It is easier to treat more acute problems by performing reflexology on the hands, and more chronic problems by performing it on the feet. If you have a headache, for example, it is more useful

Treating Common Ailments of the Hands and Feet

Ailment	Remedy
Psoriasis	1 cup Dead Sea mud
Fungus	5 drops (total) lavender, patchouli, and/or tea tree essential oil
Stress	5 drops (total) lavender and/or marjoram essential oil *or* 10 drops Rescue Remedy (Bach Flower Remedy
Fatigue	5 drops (total) peppermint, ginger, and/or orange blossom essential oil
Negative Energy	1 cup vinegar or 5 drops cedar oil essential or 5 drops of cedar essential oil added to a shallow basin of water.

Soak hands or feet for 5–10 minutes.

to treat it by applying pressure to the corresponding reflex in your hand, rather than in your foot. If you have headaches all the time, you want to work through the feet.

You can perform reflexology on yourself, but it's easier to have a partner do it for you.

Use the accompanying reflexology charts from the Laura Norman Reflexology Center and Spa, New York, New York, to understand the points on your hands and feet that correspond to the rest of your body

THE HANDS

Although reflexology can be applied to both hands and feet, the two extremities are quite different from one another. For instance, it often takes less time and effort to work with the hands than it does with the feet.

The great yogis taught that our hands held minor versions of the larger spinal chakras in them, so we can tap into different sorts of energy with our hands. Hands can be read, to tell your past, present, and future. Your nail beds can tell a thing or two about your physical health; when you're in the hospital, they remove your nail polish to check the color of the moons in your nail beds to see if oxygen is reaching your extremities—a bluish tinge can mean trouble.

Hands are also the tools of loving touch. Think of how a mother can so easily calm her baby by gently running her hands over its arms, or how a kind touch from a lover can reawaken your spirit. Keep in mind, the backs of the hands need to be treated gently as well. Certain nerve endings are very close to the surface, and too deep a touch can lead to feelings of anxiety.

Hands-On Smoother

FROM BODY, MIND AND SPIRIT, WESTPORT, CONNECTICUT

Body, Mind and Spirit is a small, personal, and charming spa that offers deeply healing body and facial treatments. They provide a small island of peace and serenity in a busy, creative town, home to many famous artists, actors, musicians, and businesspeople. The spa also has a wonderful gift shop, with lots of home spa supplies available.

6 drops tangerine essential oil
4 drops lavender essential oil
2 drops tea tree essential oil
¼ cup sea salts (fine)

Blend the essential oils. Mix together with sea salt (if mixture is too thick, add lukewarm water).

Give yourself a mini-massage on your hands, using small circular movements over joints, wrists, and knuckles. Use your thumb and forefinger between each finger and your thumb and a circular motion over the palm of your hand. The point between your thumb and forefinger represents your large intestines. Increasing its flow is beneficial in releasing toxins. Press into the fleshy mound next to the bone indentation. Rub firmly to release endorphins and release pain. Concentrate on the hand that is most sensitive. Alternatively, press and hold to help with constipation. Repeat on your other hand. This may also relieve any tension in your neck or head. Breathe as you massage to also help increase oxygen flow into your bloodstream.

Use a gentle circular motion on your fingertips and especially over nail bed and cuticle area.

Tea tree is antifungal and antibacterial and lavender is aromatic and relaxing and helps soothe our senses. The massage improves circulation, which also increases blood flow and, therefore, stimulates the body's natural defense system.

THE EXECUTIVE STRESS BATH
FOR THE HANDS

The spa experience needn't be strictly limited to your home, or to time spent in your bathrobe. You can even rejuvenate yourself in your office, in the middle of the day. The Executive Stress Bath consists of a small bowl of warm water and three to six drops of an essential oil.

- Choose calming oils like lavender or chamomile if it's a little relaxing tension relief you're after.
- Use invigorating oils like peppermint or eucalyptus if you need a quick pick-me-up.
- Make lemon/lavender, ginger/nutmeg, or orange/juniper combinations for mind-clearing.
- Combining rosemary and cedar creates a nerve tonic and brain stimulant that helps you release negativity.

Hand and Foot Plant Baths

FROM THE CENTRE DE CURES MESSAGUE-PHYTOTHERM

CRANS-MONTANA, SWITZERLAND

Located in the heart of the Swiss Alps, the Crans-Montana affords visitors a magnificent panoramic view. Situated in the sunniest region in Switzerland, this spa is like a true Garden of Eden.

The Crans-Montana Spa is committed to the healing powers of plants, using treatments in keeping with those used years ago by Maurice Messague, a world-famous French herbalist who treated his clients with herbs and footbaths. His impressive list of followers included Churchill and Stalin.

I would recommend doing this hand and footbath on a regular basis. It is detoxifying, and it improves blood circulation and stimulation of the internal organs.

½ cup of each of the following plant extracts: (or as many as are available)

Celandine
Ground ivy
Graminis radix
Stinging nettle
Rosemary
Buckthorn
Lime blossom

Mix the extracts. Boil two quarts water, and add to it 1 cup of the extract mixture. Before each bath, warm this mixture up again without boiling and without adding more water.

In the mornings, enjoy a tepid footbath lasting six to ten minutes.

In the evenings give yourself a hand bath, as warm as possible, lasting six to ten minutes.

This mixture will last for sixteen baths. After the last bath, throw the rest of the mixture away.

THE FEET

In many cultures, the feet are believed to be sacred. Muslims wash their feet in special tubs before entering a mosque. Jesus is said to have had his feet anointed by his mother, Mary. Royalty have been known to have their subjects kiss their feet.

The feet are quite special. Just like the hands, they can be read, too, for your past, present, and future. You can also tell what is going on throughout the rest of your body by noticing the condition of your feet near certain reflex points. Calluses in certain areas can be indications of medical or emotional issues. In fact, there are doctors who can do complete diagnostics of the body and psyche through the feet.

The Ground You Walk On

Feeling stressed at work? Here's a break you can take that's better than coffee. If you're wearing knee-highs or socks, and you work in an area where it isn't all concrete, you can go for a walk outside— barefoot. Just a short walk will do. You'll notice that it will make all the difference in the rest of your day.

The Portuguese Toe Massage

You are getting sleepy. . . . I learned this massage technique from a friend of mine, whose mother was a famous Portuguese artist. It had me sound asleep in minutes. It's a quick and easy way for you and your partner to help each other relax. One can do it to the other, or you can perform it on each other simultaneously.

With your partner in a relaxed and comfortable position, take one foot with both hands and gently massage each toe for one to two minutes. There are reflex points for the brain, eyes, and sinuses in the toes, and so this massage will have your partner sleeping like a baby. There's no right or wrong way to do this massage. Use your intuition, and listen to your partner.

The feet are very sensitive. They release negative energy, but they also absorb positive energy—and a whole lot more. The feet, with their large pores, are highly absorbent. So you can treat the whole body with salts and essential oils just by soaking the feet. If you're at all skeptical, try this: rub a cut clove of garlic on the soles of your feet. Within fifteen minutes, that garlic will travel up your body, and you will have garlic breath!

If you don't have time to soak your feet in a footbath, you can turn your shower into a footbath in the morning by closing the drain and putting sea salt and essential oils into the tub. Negative energy will be released, and the aromatic, healing essences will be absorbed.

One of the best therapies for releasing negative feelings and energy is to walk barefoot outside. There, your feet will connect with the energies of the earth. You become grounded. Even better is to walk along the shore, cleansing your feet in the salty seawater.

Aromatherapy Footbath

FROM THE MANDARA SPA AT THE CHEDI, UBUD, GIANYAR, BALI

Perched high up on the edge of a rich, green river valley in Bali's central foothills is this tranquil and secluded hillside retreat. All the treatments are given in a spa villa with a beautiful garden, its own pool, and a reflecting pond.

All Mandara Spa combination packages begin with an Aromatherapy Floral Footbath. In Balinese culture, foot washing symbolizes a cleansing of the soul. The flowers represent the essence of nature, and serve to add beauty to the ritual.

3 drops lavender, peppermint, or lemongrass essential oil

A handful of fresh flowers, either from your garden or a flower shop
   (roses or tropical flowers are great)

Saltwater from the ocean, or tap water with added sea salt

Fill a footbath with enough saltwater to cover feet. Add your favorite flowers and essential oil.

Begin by gently massaging the feet.

Wash the feet with soap and a soft brush.

Afterwards, slough rough skin with a volcanic pumice stone, which you can find in any drugstore. Dry the feet with a towel. Refresh with a spray of 2 oz. water and ten drops of lavender oil.

SEA SALT FOOTBATH

1 bucket of water (or sit on the edge of your tub)

1 cup sea salt

They have bath chairs for the tub at pharmacies—usually used for bathing the elderly—and some even have a back to them.

Add sea salt to the bucket of water (or to two to three inches of water in the tub). Immerse feet for five to twenty minutes.

For a really authentic experience, you can also sip your favorite "beach drink" and play the Beach Boys and let yourself slip into a different state of mind while the sea salts drain out the bad vibrations circulating around in your body!

Walking on Water

Footbaths are among the easiest spa treatments to enjoy, and they're so rejuvenative. All you need is a basin or bucket full of warm water and some essential oils.

Some guidelines: For perspiring feet, use three drops clary, four drops cypress, and three drops lavender. For tired, aching feet, use five drops juniper, three drops lavender, and two drops rosemary.

MUD FOOTBATH

If you suffer from dry, scaly skin, eczema, or psoriasis, this soak is therapeutic and curative. This is also a great treatment for winter's dry itchy legs!

> 1 cup Dead Sea mud
> Essential oil of your choice
> Body lotion or oil

Rub wet mud on legs from the knees down.

Soak for twenty minutes in a bucket of water to which you have added the rest of the mud and a few drops of your essential oil.

Remove the mud with a loofah to exfoliate the dead skin.

Apply Body Lotion

Power of Touch for Tired Feet

FROM BODY, MIND AND SPIRIT,
WESTPORT, CONNECTICUT

6–12 drops peppermint essential oil
4 drops tea tree essential oil
2 tablespoons pure vegetable oil

Blend essential oils and mix with vegetable oil.

As you massage your feet with the oils, place your thumb between the bones leading to your big toe and the second toe. Slide up between the bones until you find the point that may be sensitive just before the bones join. This point is your liver point. Press deeply between the bones into this area and slowly breathe out, slow and long. Now use circular motions, especially around each cuticle and nail bed. Use your thumb on the bottom of your foot, holding and supporting it with both hands. Let both thumbs glide up your foot through the center until you can locate a point in the middle just below the pad of your joint of the big toe. This is your kidney point. Again press deeply and breathe out, slow and long. This flow of breath is used to increase your energy flow, and the peppermint oil has the property of stimulating blood flow and decreasing any muscle cramping and/or spasm. Repeat on the other foot.

Note: The feet are very quick to absorb oils because they have large pores. Therefore three to six drops of the oil mixture per foot is adequate to experience the feeling of peace, relaxation, and/or energy.

QUICKIE:
Healing Athlete's Foot

Here's a quick remedy for athlete's foot. Honey is a natural skin softener. Lavender and tea tree oils are anti-fungal.

½ cup honey
5 drops lavender or tea tree essential oil

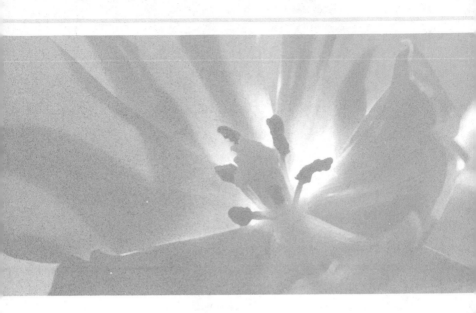

CHAPTER EIGHT

Soulful Retreats

*I*n many cultures around the world, spa treatments are designed for spiritual benefits as much as physical. In fact, there are treatments that are more spiritually focused than anything else; they are believed to heal the body and the mind by way of the spirit. There are others that combine physical and spiritual elements.

Meditation, for example, incorporating positive affirmations and mantras, can be especially effective while you're bathing in water infused with fragrant essential oils. The bath and oils relax the body and mind, and open the unconscious. Focus on an important goal in this setting, and it can easily be manifested as a reality. At the same time, your skin and organs are benefiting from a detoxifying and nourishing soak in a bath of essential oils.

Many of the ritual-oriented treatments in this chapter have

been practiced for ages, and continue to be handed down to new generations for their subtle but effective healing powers. Others are modern adaptations based on ancient wisdom.

WHAT YOU BELIEVE

Regardless of your particular personal beliefs, you have a spirit. In this chapter, I present ways of connecting with and nurturing that spirit which may be new to you. It is important to note that none of the ideas put forth in this chapter conflict with any religion or faith. They are based on principles of universal energy, which are shared among several cultures. The ancient Chinese,

Meditation's Many Benefits

Christopher Stopa, Transcendental Meditation teacher and energy field healer, explains meditation as a method by which to calm the mind, and to settle the body and spirit into a state of maximum rest. Meditation releases stress. Stress, as we know, is a major factor in the aging process. People who meditate regularly suffer fewer illnesses, have more energy, have faster reaction times to stimuli, have more stamina, and reflect less stress on their faces and bodies. There are many methods of meditation. Releasing stress on a regular basis allows the inner beauty of a person to rise to the surface, creating an outer glow of peace and serenity.

Indian, Egyptian, Jewish, Aztec, Celtic, and Japanese cultures, among others, all had very similar concepts of energy and the mind/body/spirit connection. For example, there are variations on the Hindu chakra systems, which appear in the both Jewish Kabballah and ancient Mayan texts. This early global commonality, at a time when people didn't travel around the world, is testament to the intrinsic validity of those ideas and these treatments.

Relaxing Meditation

FROM THE KALANI OCEANSIDE RESORT RETREAT, HAWAII

At the resort, Kathy Elder offers this relaxation technique used in her Restorative Yoga class. She suggests enhancing your relaxation by using a lavender-scented eye pillow. "Conscious relaxation initiates a balanced and healthy life. We know in yoga that if we are breathing erratically we are thinking erratically."

1. Count to yourself rhythmically 500, 501, 502 on each inhalation and exhalation, so that each breath is the same duration.
2. Observe the quality of the breath as it moves silkily through the nostrils. With every inhalation we nourish ourselves; with every exhalation we cleanse ourselves.
3. Continue conscious breathing and conscious counting for approximately five minutes.

4. Stop counting. Rest for three or four breaths.
5. In addition to counting the duration of the inhalation and exhalation, count silently the number of breaths you take. Example: Inhale, exhale, think "one"; inhale, exhale, think "two."
6. Constantly remember the quality and the motion of the breath in the body. Let every exhalation generate a sense of release.
7. When you get to ten breaths, once again stop counting and take three or four resting breaths.
8. Start again.

If you forget where you are, just give yourself a little inner smile and start from the beginning. After two rounds stop counting and let the breath regulate itself. Uncover the eyes. Leave the eyes closed for several breaths, and when you are ready, let the eyes open gently.

MEDITATION 101

Meditation is one of the most common spiritual practices used in religions and belief systems throughout the world. It is also very popular at spas because it is such a key to health and beauty. Spas today have special rooms set aside for meditation, and they often hold meditation retreats.

Meditation is one of the greatest beauty secrets. When you meditate, you relax the muscles of the face. Look into the faces of monks and you will see great youthfulness. Because meditation reduces stress, it helps to keep cells from breaking down as quickly as they might. It also helps to activate the pituitary gland, which maintains hormonal balance.

Meditation can be a simple practice, but it is often mistakenly thought to be very complicated and difficult. There are many different variations and approaches to meditation, yet it is something everyone can do and benefit from in many ways. Meditation alone can be its own practice, it can be part of a treatment, or it can be a state of mind you achieve at any time by being mindful of the truth you are hearing internally, and tuning out what is happening externally.

Very simply, meditation is the absence of thought. It is a tuning out of all outside noise so that you can awaken to your internal voice. It is the quieting of the conscious mind so that the subconscious can hear and be heard. It is the opposite of prayer; when we pray, we speak to God or divine spirits but when we meditate, we listen to the divine within us. In a meditative state, we become receptive to spiritual energies, to wisdom, and to positive energy, which enters our bodies through the crown chakra.

One of the beauties of meditation is that it requires very little in order to practice it. The yogis in the Himalayas used to go into the caves there and bring little with them. They would find a piece of charcoal, draw a black dot on the cave wall, and then focus on that dot as a way of entering a meditative state. In the absence of a piece of charcoal, they would stare at one of their thumbnails.

THE POWER OF SUGGESTION

When we enter a meditative state, we open the subconscious part of the mind—the part of the mind that is open to suggestion. This is wonderful for helping us to adopt new attitudes and achieve our goals.

There are two tools we can use in a meditative state to encourage us to move in a positive direction: creative visualization and affirmations.

Creative visualization is one notch above daydreaming. In order to use it most effectively, you imagine what you want—to do, or to have—*as if you already have it*. Once your mind is convinced that you already have it, you will believe that you *can* have it, and will therefore be more likely to get it.

Affirmations are simply positive statements you tell yourself. You can reinforce self-love this way, with statements like, "I love you, [your name], and I always will," and "I know my beauty." You can also encourage yourself, with affirmations like, "I will finish writing my book," or "I deserve to be healthy." Your subconscious believes whatever you tell it, so be sure to say only the most positive things. Remember: the key components to beauty are self-acceptance and self-love.

Self-Remembering: A 30-Minute Relaxation Meditation

FROM THE DIRECTOR OF THE MANDARA SPA
AT THE ROYAL GARDEN RESORT, HUA HIN, THAILAND

Tangkis, a spa manager and trainer, has been a serious student of meditation for over twenty years. His guru, a 105-year-old Balinese master, is his guide and inspiration for training the therapists at the spa.

1. Sit in any way that you are most comfortable.
2. Close your eyes and relax.
3. Take a normal breath and exhale strongly. Repeat three to five times until you feel your whole body relax.
4. Start to take a normal breath but breathe into your head through your face (as though you are facing the wind). As you exhale, bring your attention to your face and head and acknowledge yourself.
5. With the next exhalation, bring the energy from your head down your neck through your right arm. Repeat, bringing the energy through your left arm.
6. From the upper body, bring your attention on the exhale down your spine past the heart, lungs, liver, kidney, stomach, and navel, to the base of the spine.
7. From your right groin take the energy down the right leg through the toes.
8. Repeat with the left leg.
9. Take one more breath and, on the exhale, acknowledge your self (your being).
10. Breathe naturally as you acknowledge everyone you have loved, starting with your parents and ending with this universe. You will feel your being expand to encompass everyone and everything that you love.
11. Sit quietly with this experience as you focus your attention on your sixth chakra (third eye).

SURRENDER TO THE UNIVERSAL LAW

This is another message from Tangkis, a spa manager and trainer. He says we must all surrender to the Universal Law.

"Most of us don't realize that we are subject to an unseen power that rules the universe. We are all trying to conquer or control everything in our lives and win every battle.

"Ask yourself: was everything that you did in the last sixty minutes a result of your will?

"Do you realize that throughout your life you experience the fluctuation of extremes—day and night, good and bad, happiness and unhappiness?

"We are stuck trying to have the best of these two worlds, but we don't realize that we are not in a position to choose. We are only a drop of water in the ocean. Why continue to struggle? Open your heart and accept life as it is. If you can accept both extremes as a natural part of life, you will be in a state of harmony."

THE THIRD EYE

The third eye chakra, located just above and between our eyebrows, provides us with the vision of our lives—but only if we are able to tune in to this chakra, and open it. We have so much more mental and psychic ability than most of us are aware of. We can build our awareness and our intuitiveness by working on opening and awakening the third eye chakra.

Here's a meditation exercise you can try:

1. Light a candle, and stare at the flame through relaxed, half-mast eyes.
2. Slow your breath, and get a good rhythm going.
3. When your eyes get tired, close them, and you'll see the flame still in your mind.

4. Do this for a few minutes, take a break, and then repeat for a little bit longer.

Try this exercise in the bathtub, and you will magnetize the water with your positive intentions. This will help you to achieve the goals you identify with your newly developed intuition.

Empty Bowl Meditation

FROM THE AYURVEDIC INSTITUTE, ALBUQUERQUE, NEW MEXICO

In Sanskrit, ayurveda *means "the Science of Life." It is an ancient system of healing developed to prevent disease, preserve health, and promote longevity.*

The mission of the Ayurvedic Institute is "the integration of the universal principles of Ayurveda with those of modern medicine, yoga, other healing disciplines, and with the individual Self to bring about total health, awareness, and harmony."

Sit comfortably and quietly with palms placed on the knees, up and open, like empty bowls. Open the mouth slightly and touch your tongue to the roof of your mouth, behind the front teeth. Pay attention to the breath. Let the lungs breathe with no effort on your part. Breath is the object of awareness. Simply watch the movement of your breath. As you are watching the movement of your breath, pay attention to the tip of your nose. Just be aware of the touch of air going into the nose. Cool air going in, warm air coming out. Sit this way quietly, observing breath, for about five minutes.

After five minutes, follow the breath. Go with the air into the nose, throat, heart, diaphragm, deep down into the belly behind the belly button, where you will experience a natural stop. Stay in this stop mode for a fraction of a second, then follow the breath on exhalation, as it reverses its course up from the belly behind the diaphragm, heart, throat, out through the nose, and out of the body to about nine inches below the nose to a second stop.

The first stop is behind the belly button; the second stop is outside the body in space. At these two stops, your breath stops. At these two stops, time stops. Movement of the breath is time. In these two stops, only existence is present. In these two stops, you are surrounded by peace and love. In these stops, God is present. In these stops, you become like an empty bowl. The moment you become like an empty bowl, the divine lips can touch you. God will seek you and pour benediction into you. Let the lungs breathe and you become the empty bowl. Practice this meditation for fifteen minutes in the morning and in the evening. As you practice this meditation, over the days, weeks, and months, you will find your time in the stops naturally prolonging until eventually inner and outer will merge at the third eye and everything will happen within you.

You may also practice this meditation in a prone position.

A BEAUTY SECRET

Gerie Bauer, of Great Spas of the World in New York, is a spa guru and consultant who has traveled around the world sitting at the feet of the masters, learning the secrets of health and beauty. She says that one of the most overlooked beauty secrets is sleep. Here she gives her advice:

"Many people can't sleep because they rethink their day or plan the next one. This tends to invigorate the mind and thus defeats the aim of relaxing in order to go to sleep. Here's a mental trick that can be used to go to sleep at night: Close your eyes and picture a black screen. White will invigorate, black tends to settle the mind down. Focus strongly on that black screen and make a definite effort not to allow a single thought to cross it. As one does you blank it out to focus on the black. Then start fuzzying away at the edges, gently and softly. Eventually you will relax your mind and go to sleep."

It also helps to have a soothing aromatherapy fragrance either in your pillow or next to the bed. Everyone reacts differently to fragrance. It should be one you have already noted to be relaxing for you. Lavender is the most commonly used essential oil for relaxation. But if you find it unappealing, try rose, chamomile, marjoram, or sandalwood.

THE SCIENCE OF SPIRITUALITY

Believe it or not, there is a lot of science behind spirituality. We are beings made of pure energy from a divine source—complex arrangements of molecules and atoms vibrating in the form of flesh and bone. While there is a great deal of mystery and mysticism surrounding the spiritual world, there are some things that are very explainable, in terms of electromagnetic energy.

Electromagnetic energy affects us at all levels—body, mind, and spirit. We all have different vibrational frequencies, meaning that our particular molecules vibrate at a unique rate. We each also have a range within which our vibrational frequency changes, depending on how we're feeling and what we're experiencing. If you have jet lag, for instance, your frequency dips. If you've had too much caffeine, your frequency is spiked. If you're in perfect harmony with yourself, your vibrations are well balanced and you're "grounded."

You may have heard the term *vibrational medicine.* This includes modalities like aromatherapy, Bach Flower Remedies, homeopathy, color therapy, and music therapy.

Because there are many dimensions to our beings, they need to be integrated in order for us to feel in a state of grace and beauty. We can do things to alter our vibrational frequencies, like meditating or practicing grounding breathing. By altering the frequency of one aspect of your being, say, your mind, you automatically affect the other aspects of your being, your body and spirit.

BRAZILIAN SHAMAN'S EMPOWERMENT RITUAL

Power objects are used in all shamanistic cultures for protection and personal empowerment. If you feel you need to shield yourself from negative energy, create your own power stone with the following steps, given to me by a shaman trained by American and Amazonian Indians. Crystals have a long tradition of use in indigenous cultures. The Mayan Indians claimed to use them to travel out of body. They believed the crystal would protect them along the way.

1. Find a quartz crystal that you like. A finger-length one with a single point would be a good choice.
2. Bury the crystal in the earth for two days. If you're a city dweller, bury it in a flowerpot.
3. Remove from the soil and soak in a glass or ceramic bowl of water for seven days. (Changing the water is optional.)

4. Wrap your crystal in plastic wrap and put it in the freezer for seven days. Your crystal is now ready for use.
5. Find a "chalice" (a wineglass will do), and put some sand from the beach in it (if not available, you can improvise).
6. Insert quartz into the sand with the point sticking up. Keep it in the chalice when you don't have it with you.
7. You now have consecrated your power stone. Use it whenever you need protection. It's best to carry it in your pocket or you can sleep with it next to your bed.

YOUR AURA

Your electromagnetic vibrations are not just in your body but around you, in what is known as your aura. In polarity therapy, it's known as your electromagnetic field, and in Chinese medicine and acupuncture, it's defined in terms of currents and meridians. These modalities are designed to help keep positive energy flowing, unobstructed, through the mind, body, and spirit. It is when this energy flows freely that our aura is intact, and we are healthy and radiant. In fact, the ancient yogis said that if your energy is flowing freely, absolutely no disease can exist within you.

You know when you just meet someone and you get certain "vibes" from them, good or bad, before you've even talked? You are sensing their aura. It is as simple as this: When your energy is free, and your aura is at its best, there is a magnetic electricity about you that attracts people to you; when you are depressed or unhappy, there is a negative current in your aura that repels people.

The aura is not just some esoteric high concept; it can be photographed by a special camera. The dominant color indicates your vibrational frequency. If you take different pictures in different moods, you'll notice that the colors surrounding you will change.

When the auric field is weak, we are vulnerable to illness. In fact, there are aura healers and energy balancers who specialize in working on keeping this electromagnetic field strong, intact, and complete—not to mention acupuncturists, polarity therapists, and reiki masters.

Your emotional and spiritual states are manifested physically. And nowhere is this more relevant than with regard to beauty. In order for the physical being to reflect beauty, the inner being needs

Angelspeak: Listening to Guidance

Trudy Griswald and I met while doing book signings at a spa. We had an instant connection and talked all night. We didn't get many books signed but we became great friends. Trudy has taught classes on talking with our angels at spas across the country and has coauthored four books on angels. She says:

"Life has become a whole lot easier since I began speaking with my angels! Your angels want to connect with you even more than you want to connect with them. Angels are always with you helping you with anything in your life you'd like to have, do, or be. Continue to call upon them each day and ask them to be with you, believe they will be there, and then let go and allow them to bring to you the right people, circumstances, and events into your life. And always say thank you. An attitude of gratitude will truly make a difference in your life."

Speaking with your angels is easier than you can believe. Here are four simple steps to follow, which we have named the "four fundamentals for living a fulfilled spiritual life." They have worked for thousands of people.

1. **Ask . . .** your angels to be with you by saying a prayer to wrap yourself in the loving light of God. Sit quietly with paper and pencil in hand. Be open and allow this very special exchange of loving energy to come through to you. Breathe deeply and relax but do not meditate.

2. **Believe and trust . . .** that your angels are with you and that you will receive a message. Let it happen. You are being guided although you may feel you are making it up. Acceptance is most important.

3. **Let go . . .** And begin writing what you know to write. Let the angels' energy or vibration come through to you whether in the form of a small soft whisper, a picture in your mind, or a feeling of knowing. The angels have the same loving voice you have heard many times before. The harder you think, the less flow there will be. As you practice receiving their dictated messages, you will hear words of comfort and guidance.

4. **Say thank you . . .** You have received a spiritual gift for which you didn't have to do anything. Simply be grateful for what you have received and acknowledge receiving it by giving thanks.

Ask questions. Expect answers. Don't complicate the process. Ask, believe, let go, and say thank you. Don't forget to ask for the name of the angel who is communicating with you. Keep practicing, as your angelic communications will come easier over time.

Negative energy is all around us. We can feel attacked by negative people or negative situations that we encounter during the day. Here is a quick and easy way to restore our power and inner harmony:

Sitting or standing, place your palms together with tips of fingers pointing downward. Vigorously rub palms together for two to three minutes or until you feel a sense of relief.

If you want, visualize the negative energy being pulled out of you and grounded into the earth.

Feel free to do this exercise anywhere, anytime. It only takes a couple of minutes and you will feel your equilibrium restored.

to be in a state of harmony, to have a strong auric field. There needs to be a core focus of inner peace and wellness.

How can you strengthen your auric field? Meditation is one very helpful way. When you meditate, the auric field becomes stronger, more dynamic, and impenetrable to negative energy and disease. Treating yourself with self-love—whether it's just basic acceptance of yourself or making time for spa treatments at home—is another aura-strengthener.

Here's a breathing exercise that is a great way to strengthen the aura and give it a positive magnetic charge, before a date, an important meeting, or any time you need to be at your best:

1. Inhale slowly, for a count of seven, imagining that you are taking that breath into the auric field above and around you.
2. Hold your breath for a count of seven, imagining that your aura is being strengthened and magnetized.
3. Exhale slowly, for seven counts.
4. Repeat this five times.

CHAKRA GUIDED MEDITATION

Consider reading this softly into a tape recorder and playing it back once you are in a comfortable position. Turn off your phones, and relax into this powerful, transformational meditation.

When you are obsessively thinking negative thoughts or experiencing negative emotions, the simplest antidote is to contemplate their opposites for at least two minutes. For example:

Anger	Peace
Frustration	Harmony
Abandonment	Security

Take a deep breath and imagine the breath you take in is an illuminating white light. Breathe this light in deeply, hold the light, and feel it circulate throughout your body. Now exhale and project the breath of light out, allowing this light to surround you. This breath of light is enfolding you in a radiant layer of protection and awakening your chakras. Breathe in, circulate the light, and breathe out. Breathe in again, circulate the light, and breathe out. Once more, breathe in, circulate the light, and breathe out.

Now become aware of and focus on the base of your spine—the very tip of your spine. Imagine the area is like a lung, inhaling and exhaling. This is your first chakra, your root chakra. Gently move your awareness there. Visualize the color red. Breathe into your root chakra the fire and energy of this red light. Imagine your root chakra is pulsating. As it's beginning to pulsate, continue to breathe in the color red. Red gives you courage and fire and aliveness. The root chakra connects you to the earth. As you continue to breathe, feel the energy of your root chakra awaken. Breathe in this courage, fire, and aliveness from this red energy. As thoughts enter your mind, ignore them. Focus on the sensations in your body. Let everything else drift away.

Now move this energy gently up your spine to the area that is two inches below your navel. This is the area of your second chakra, your sacral chakra. There is a great deal of energy here for sexuality, for healing of the body, and for the creation of life. Visualize the color orange and bring that wonderful, pulsating orange into your sacral chakra. Let this orange spread through your entire pelvic area, dissolving any blocks, any fears, any tensions, and any anxieties in your life. We hold a great many negative emotions here. Allow the orange light to purify and transform your emotions. Feel yourself bathed in this vibrant orange light. As you inhale and exhale, activate your power to create, your power to transform.

With your next breath, move your awareness up your spinal cord to the center of your body at the navel. This chakra is called the solar plexus. Visualize a radiant golden sun that's filled with energy and power and vibrancy. The energy of the sun is constant. Nothing daunts this power; nothing can diminish it. I want you to become a source of undiminished light and power. Nothing can take your power away. You are strong. You are a golden light. Use your breathing to fill your solar plexus with light and energy. Breathe the light all the way into your abdomen and expand it as fully as possible. Exhale. Inhale again, breathing the golden light into your abdomen, and exhale. Once more, breathe in this light, expand your abdomen, and exhale. Now I want you to visualize yourself as a great vibrant sun, a source of power and energy. Experience the peace that comes with this power. You have the power to accomplish what is necessary for your highest good, what is necessary for your soul's fulfillment in this life. You have the power for success and happiness. You have the power to live in harmony and prosperity. You have the power to achieve inner peace. As you are breathing into this chakra, feel yourself existing right now in a state of total fulfillment in this lifetime.

Move your energy, following your spinal cord up to the center of your chest. This is the heart chakra. Visualize a beautiful pink light emanating from the center of your chest. Let your heart circulate acceptance, peace, and unconditional love. Breathe this pink light into your heart, and as you breathe, let the energy of love remove your insecurities and replace them with contentment. Let this unconditional love wash away self-doubt and self-criticisms. Breathe in the pink light until you are in harmony with your soul. In this state of self-love, you can communicate with your soul and ask it anything you wish to know. Ask it the questions that most concern you in your life. Ask your soul to tell you about your mission in life, the path for you to take. Once you have asked, sit in absolute silence. Do not allow any thoughts to enter, and do not contemplate any answers you may get.

With your next breath, move your energy up your spine through each of your chakras, from the root through the sacral, through your solar plexus and your heart into the throat chakra. Concentrate on the point behind your throat on your spine on the back of your neck. This is the chakra of creative expression. This is where great works are expressed—music, art, poetry. This is from where your soul speaks. Visualize blue, the color of the heavens. Breathe in this blue light and energy through your throat chakra. Inhale and exhale the blue energy. Let your throat expand, let it fill with the colors and vastness of the sky. The place from which you speak your truth is expanding. This is the chakra through which you will manifest expressions from the higher realms, from the angels, from your spirit guides. Feel yourself in a state of rest and peace and openness. You are now a perfect channel of divine will, divine light, and divine expression. Experience the infinity of the heavens, and listen to the celestial voices of the angels.

To take your energy higher, breathe deeply and move all of your awakened energy as a fountain up through your body. Feel the tingling in your spine. Bring that energy to the point between and slightly above your eyebrows. This is your third eye chakra. Visualize a brilliant purple light. Inhale and exhale this purple light into your third eye. Continue to inhale and exhale this purple light, and as you do, you are awakening your insight, your wisdom, your intuition. Inside the purple there is a blue pearl of wisdom. I want you to concentrate, look inside your third eye, and look for this blue pearl of wisdom, of enlightenment, of inner vision. This is the chakra where your sight is awakened, your inner sight, the sight to see the past and the future, the inner sight to see truth. Continue to breathe in the powerful purple light to expand your vision beyond this world. You want to expand your vision beyond what your mind perceives. Let yourself be bathed in the purple light and look for the blue pearl inside your third eye. Relax and breathe gently as you do this. Enjoy the expansion of your perceptions.

Once again, you are going to breathe in and move your energy and light up through the chakras until you reach the top of your head. At the very center of the top of your head is the crown chakra. This is the chakra that joins your spiritual self with your human self. Here lives your idealism and your higher self. As you inhale and exhale, imagine there's a beautiful lotus flower of many petals. These petals are open wide as if in a state of receiving. Imagine these petals vibrating a cosmic white light—the light is alive, the light dances, the light has movement. This white light is a waterfall flowing from the sky, from the infinite consciousness into your crown chakra and moving through your entire body. As you breathe, celebrate yourself in this brilliant waterfall of light. It's washing you; it's purifying you. Every cell of your being is being purified by this white light. You are being healed by this light. As you breathe in and out, this waterfall of light is washing, purifying the energies around you. It is expanding into your auric field, protecting you, nourishing you, creating a dynamic force field around you. You are a being of light; you are the wisdom of God. This is your spiritual center of truth. Quietly meditate and allow this white light to transform you.

Now, walk through life radiating your inner strength and beauty.

Sea salts and muds

Frontier Herbs
3021 78th Street
Norway, IA 52318
800-669-3275

Neptune's Gift
Pinnacle Minerals Inc.
2241 Speers Avenue
Saskatoon, SK, Canada S7L 5X6
800-749-7158

Utama Spice
P.T. Supa Dupa Spice
P.O. Box 81
Ubud, Bali 80571
Indonesia
Tel 62361-975051
Fax 62361-974865

Water Magic
20 Crooked Mile Road
Westport, CT 06880
800-331-8854
www.watermagic.com
Also at health food stores, spa gift shops, and pharmacies

Essential oils
Aura Cacia
P.O. Box 399
Weaverville, CA 96093
800-437-3301

Aromaland Inc.
Route 20
Box 29AL
Santa Fe, NM 87507
800-933-5257

Aroma Vera
5901 Rodeo Drive
Los Angeles, CA 90016
800-669-9514

Pure Essentials
59 Dover Street
Patterson, NJ 07501
Tel 973-881-8220
Fax 973-881-8226
www.pureessentials.com

Utama Spice
P.T. Supa Dupa Spice
P.O. Box 81
Ubud, Bali 80571
Indonesia
Tel 62361-975051
Fax 62361-974865
Also at health food stores

Bach Flower Remedies
Nelson Bach, USA
100 Research Drive
Wilmington, MA 01887
978-988-3833
Also at health food stores

Homeopathic remedies
Boericke and Tafel, Inc.
2381 Circadian Way
Santa Rosa, CA 95407
707-571-8208
Also at health food stores

Reflexology training, sessions, books, and videos
Laura Norman and Associates
Reflexology Center and Spa
41 Park Avenue
Suite 8A
New York, NY 10016
212-532-4404
Lauranormanreflexology.com

Sponges and brushes
Pharmacies, bath and body shops, health food stores, and Spa
Boutiques

Spa travel
Great Spas of the World
International Health Spa Specialists
Gerie and Bernard Bauer
10 Park Avenue
Suite 4C
New York, NY 10016
800-SPA-TIME
212-889-8170
www.greatspas.com

Bath and body products
Water Magic, Inc.
20 Crooked Mile Road
Westport, CT 06880
800-331-8854
www.watermagic.com
Also at health food stores, spa retail shops, and pharmacies

Meditation
Angelspeak
Trudy Griswold
4680 Black Rock Turnpike
Fairfield, CT 06430
Tel 203-319-1903
Fax 203-319-9301
www.angelspeak.com

Christopher Stopa, M.S., M.F.T.
435 Newtown Turnpike
Redding, CT 06896
203-938-3187

SPA DIRECTORY

Arogya Holistic Healing
131 Post Road East
Westport, CT 06880
Tel 203-226-2682
Fax 203-222-8190
A holistic spa offering authentic healing treatments such as qi gong
and Chinese herbal therapy in a soothing, nurturing environment.

Arte Salon
284 Lafayette Street
New York, NY 10012
Tel 212-941-5932
Fax 212-941-8577
Located in SoHo, Manhattan, the salon offers aromatherapeutic salon
services.
A good resource for Mixd Flava shea butter products.

Ayurvedic Institute
11311 Menaul Boulevard N.E.
Albuquerque, NM 87112
Tel 505-291-9698
Fax 505-294-7572
www.ayurveda.com
Recognized as one of the leading Ayurvedic health spas outside of
India, established to teach traditional therapy of East Indian
Ayurvedic, including herbs, nutrition, yoga, and acupressure massage.

Body, Mind and Spirit
1799 Post Road.
Westport, CT 06880
Tel 203-254-7721
Fax 203-254-7783
This spa's focus is on healing the body, mind, and spirit. The owner,
Lisa West, is an R.N. who is dedicated to helping clients achieve
inner peace.

Centre De Cures Messague-Phytotherm
Hotel Crans-Montana
Case Postale 372
CH 3962 Crans-Montana, Switzerland
Tel 41(0)2748504-44
www.crans-montana.ch
Phytotherm, practiced here, is a plant-based therapy whose
philosophy is that prevention is of paramount importance to staying
in good health and feeling young to an advanced age.

Chiva-Som
73/4 Petchkasem Road
Hva Hin 77110
Thailand
Tel (66) 32536536
Fax (66) 32511154
www.Chivasom.net
As one of the leading health resorts in the world, Chiva-Som won the
Conde Nast traveler's award for the best overseas spa. This "Haven of
Life" is a true elixir for rejuvenation of body and soul.

The Datai
Teluk Datai Pulau Langkawi
Kedah Darul Aman, Malaysia 070001
Tel (011) 60-4-9592500
Fax (011) 60-4-9592600
Tucked away in the middle of an ancient rain forest, the resort also
has a secluded beach facing the Andaman Sea. This natural spa
experience completely pervades all the senses.

Four Seasons Resort
Sayan Ubud Gianyar 80571
Bali, Indonesia
Tel (62) 361 977577
Fax (62) 361 977588
www.fourseasons.com/sayan
Nestled in the central highlands of Bali, the spa is influenced by the
calming influences of the Agung River. The accent is on earth
elements and the use of clays and spices combined with fresh herbs,
leaves, and flowers from the region.

Four Seasons Resort Maldives at Kuda Huraa
North Male Atoll
Republic of Maldives
Tel (960) 444-888
Fax (960) 443-388
www.fourseasons.com/maldives
This island spa is a tranquil oasis dedicated to peace, harmony, and
balance. Treatments harmonize ancient regional traditions with the
finest natural ingredients.

Hakone Prince Hotel
144 Moto-hakone Hakone-machi
Ashigarashimo-gun
Kanagawa, Japan 250-0592
Tel 0460-3-1111
Fax 0460-3-7616
www.princehotels.co.jp/hakone.e
With its magnificent scenery, Hakone is one of the most popular
places in Japan. The hotel is located on Lake Ashi, at the base of Mt.

Fuji. Its open-air hot spring has a beautiful view of the lake and is sure to soothe and revitalize body and spirit.

Hershey Spa—Hershey Resorts
100 West Chocolate Avenue
University Drive
Hershey, PA 17033
Tel 717-520-5450
www.HersheyPA.com
Therapeutic and fun, the spa's treatments focus on chocolate as a main ingredient for many of its services.

Hosteria Las Quintas Eco Spa
Blvd. Diaz Ordaz No. 9
Cantarranas, C.P. 62240
Cuernavaca, Mexico
Tel (5273) 18-2949
Fax (5273) 18-3895
www.hlasquintas.com
This spa embraces an eco-fitness concept with tours to various ecological and archeological sites. Located inside a "walled estate" featuring 100,000 square feet of lush gardens, the spa also offers a sweat lodge.

The Ibah
Tjampuhan, Ubud
Bali, Indonesia
Tel (62) 361 974466
Fax (62) 361 974467
Run by an Ubud royal family, this is an intimate and serene luxury resort and spa located on the banks of a sacred river. The emphasis is on meditation and relaxation.

Imperial Mandara Spa
Imperial Queens Park Hotel
199 Sukhumvit 22
Bangkok, Thailand 10110
Tel 662-261-9000
Fax 662-258-2327

The philosophy of this spa is that beauty is a holistic concept that embraces the inner and outer self.

Kalani Oceanside Resort
Rural Route 2
Box 4500
Pahoa, HI 96778
Tel 800-800-6886
808-965-78828 (World Wide)
www.KALANI.com
Kalani is located on the southeast coast of Hawaii, known as the "Big Island." This retreat and spa offers a lush haven for soulful retreats or exciting eco-adventures.

Lausanne Palace & Spa
7-9 rue du Grand-ChOne 1002
Lausanne, Switzerland
Tel (41-21) 331-3131
Fax (41-21) 323-2571
www.Lausanne-Palace.com
A place of extraordinary beauty and elegance. The philosophy of healing incorporates Ayurveda, Bach Flower Remedies, Qi Gong, and Thalassotherapy.

Le Meridien Nirwana
Nirwana Golf & Spa Resort
P.O. 158, Kediri
Tanah Lot 82171
Bali, Indonesia
Tel (62) 361-815900
Fax (62) 361 815901/07
www.lemeridien-bali.com.
Located on one of Bali's most sacred sites. A spiritual aura of peace and sacredness pervades the grounds and provides the setting for some of the most healing treatments in the world.

Mandara Spa at the Chedi Ubud
Gianyar 80572
Bali, Indonesia

Tel (62) 361 975963
Fax (62) 361 975968
www.chediubud@GHMhotels.com
The spa setting for treatments at the Chedi reflects the feeling
of sacredness and inner nourishment the Balinese believe can only
be obtained in the mountains, where they believe the gods
reside.

Noelle Spa for Beauty and Wellness
1100 High Ridge Road
Stamford, CT 06905
Tel 203-322-3445
Fax 203-321-1477
www.noelle.com
A premiere day spa in Connecticut offering water treatments, exotic
facials, and other European-inspired treatments.

The Oaks at Ojai Spa
122 East Ojai Avenue
Ojai, CA 93023
Tel 805-646-5573
Fax 805-640-1504
www.oaksspa.com
The Oaks offers a serene, yet upbeat atmosphere in which to get fit.
Choose from sixteen fitness classes daily, as well as hiking and biking
in the beautiful Ojai.

The Oberoi, Lombok
P.O. Box 1096
83001 Mataram
West Lombok
N.T.B. Indonesia
Tel (62-361) 730-361
Fax (62-361) 730-791
Surrounded by fishing villages and palm groves, the Oberoi nestles in
a tranquil bay. The treatments at the spa are designed to provide
indigenous and rejuvenating treatments within luxurious
surroundings.

The Palms at Palm Springs
572 North Indian Canyon Drive
Palm Springs, CA 92262
Tel 760-325-1111
Fax 760-327-0867
www.palmsspa.com
This spa offers programs on the cutting edge of fitness, while pampering its guests with spa treatments for beauty and wellness.

Rajvilas
Oberoi Hotel & Resort
Goner Road, Jaipur
Rajasasthan-303 012
India
Tel (91) 141-68-0101
Fax (91) 141-68-0202
The spa offers a complete world of health, beauty, and relaxation through what it calls "pure pampering." Its natural approach encompasses the traditional Indian Ayurvedic principles and the ancient art of aromatherapy.

The Ritz Carlton
Jalan Karang Mas Sejatera
Jimbaran, Bali 80364, Indonesia
Tel (62) 361 702 222
Fax (62) 361 701 555
www.ritzcarlton.com
A trek to a secluded Bali beach, indigenous body treatments and outdoor masages in a clifftop pavilion are just a few of the "Enliven the senses" therapies offered at this world-class spa. The treatments are designed to restore physical health and well-being.

Rosewater Spa of Oakville
156 Church Street
Oakville, ON, Canada
Tel 905-338-7724
Fax 905-338-6432
www.rosewaterspa.com
A place of serenity, offering therapeutic massage and restorative skin treatments.

Royal Garden Resort/Mandara Spa
107/1 Phetkasem Beach Road
Hua Hin, Thailand 77110
Tel (66) 32-511881
Fax (66) 32-512422
A completely natural outdoor spa located on an expansive sandy beach.

The Sanctuary Zara Spa
P.O. Box 5315
Amman, 11183, Jordan
Tel (011) 962 6 4655378
Fax (011) 962 6 4646782
www.thesanctuary.co.uk
Since ancient times, the Dead Sea, famous for its medical healing properties, has been a mecca for those in search of healing and rejuvenation. This spa offers an array of medical treatments focused on the nearby Dead Sea and its salts and muds.

The Sterling Institute Spa
402 Don Gaspar Avenue
Santa Fe, NM 87501
Tel 505-984 3223
www.thesterlinginstitute.com
This spa focuses on health and healthy living, offering a wide range of therapies and programs that heal and educate the client.

Taj Exotica
Pte Ltd, 10 Meduziyaaraiy
Magu, Male 20-05
Republic of Maldives
Tel (011) 960-444451
Fax (011) 960-445925
A secluded, peaceful island resort offering treatments in the Asian tradition and therapies that represent a global fusion of influences from Bali, Europe, Hawaii, Japan, and China.

INDEX

Page numbers in *italic* indicate illustrations, those in **bold** indicate tables.